of human behavior we are more willing to question and alter. The acceptance of new ideas of what is sexually okay is now so immediate you'd think entire generations had been holding their breath—people being born, living, and dying, yet never daring to explore their own sexuality, afraid that only she/he ever felt certain erotic desires, only he/she was aberrant and everyone else was "normal." Then, suddenly, The Word is out; without seeming to pause for even a sigh of relief, everybody knows without further discussion that it is not only okay, but that it has always been okay.

To suggest you ever questioned it is to show what a hopeless square you were to begin with. It took years for Kinsey's findings in the '40s to make their full cultural impact, but the revolution Masters and Johnson introduced in the '60s was immediately accepted as not revolutionary at all. Right away, their findings became part of everyone's workaday bedroom knowledge. "Sure, what else is new?"

Oral sex, for example. In the '50s, I almost fainted when a man suggested it. Yet I almost fainted with pleasure when he did it. Today, who would dare suggest that oral sex was bad, dirty, perverted—or even unusual?

During the five years I was compiling material for *My Secret Garden,* I could not find a doctor or psychiatrist who would intelligently discuss women's sexual fantasies. It was still a taboo subject. In 1968, before I decided to write the book, I did some research in the giant New York Public Library and the even larger British Museum library in London. In the millions upon millions of cards on file in these two vast repositories of practically everything ever written in the English language, I did not find a single book or magazine article that dealt with the subject, even though, by definition, women's sexual fantasies were of more than intellectual interest to one-half of the human race.

I spoke to at least a dozen psychiatrists in both the United States and Great Britain. The most any of these

AN INTRODUCTION

Dear Nancy:

I finished your book this morning, and all I can say is Thank God someone opened my eyes to this aspect of human sexuality while I am still young enough to be just at the beginning of my sexual life. Your book has totally changed my way of thinking. I am seventeen and until a few months ago, had had intercourse with only one person—my boyfriend for two years. Perhaps that is why I have fantasized so much during our sessions. But whatever the reason, it always made me feel guilty, unfaithful, and perverted—and I suppose this negative feeling about myself was another factor that kept me from enjoying sex with him.

Reading *My Secret Garden* has shown me in the clearest terms that sex and fantasies are not something to be endured, but to be enjoyed. Your book has chopped years off the time it would have taken me to make these discoveries myself. Thank you for allowing me to be reborn sexually before it was too late to change my beliefs, and before I got clogged down forever in sexual guilt.

Sincerely,

Mary

☐ Sexual mores and practices have shown an age-old resistance to change. Today, there is hardly any part

1

CONTENTS

"Your book *My Secret Garden* reduces women to men's sexual level."

—Dr. Theodore I. Rubin, to Nancy Friday, in NBC radio interview, 1973

"Aren't women entitled to a little lust too?"

—Nancy Friday's reply

This book belongs to the women whose letters fill it. Many wrote to question their own sexuality, others to confirm it. From them all, I have learned about my own.

—N. F.

An *Original* Publication of POCKET BOOKS

POCKET BOOKS, a division of Simon & Schuster Inc.
1230 Avenue of the Americas, New York, NY 10020

ISBN: 0-671-74102-0

First Pocket Books printing June 1975

27 26 25 24 23

POCKET and colophon are registered trademarks of
Simon & Schuster Inc.

Cover design by Designed To Print

Printed in the U.S.A.

NANCY FRIDAY

FORBIDDEN FLOWERS

MORE WOMEN'S SEXUAL FANTASIES

POCKET BOOKS

New York   London   Toronto   Sydney   Tokyo   Singapore

. **Books by Nancy Friday**

My Secret Garden: Women's Sexual Fantasies
Forbidden Flowers: More Women's Sexual Fantasies

Published by POCKET BOOKS

"All Women Have Sexual Fantasies

though sometimes they won't admit it, even to themselves. Fantasies are make-believe states used to enhance reality. A fantasy can give a woman an added sense of life and all its possibilities. It is the *unexamined* corners of the mind that breed neurosis and fear—not the portions of ourselves we know, recognize and accept."

—*Cosmopolitan*

FORBIDDEN
FLOWERS

Now we can talk about what we used to just think about. More Women's Sexual Fantasies

NANCY FRIDAY

learned men would concede was that perhaps some women did have sexual fantasies when they masturbated; otherwise, they said, the phenomenon was limited to the sexually frustrated and/or to the pathological. They took the initial fact that a woman had sexual fantasies as a sign of sickness. The idea that a happily married woman, sexually satisfied by a beloved husband, might still have erotic pictures in mind—perhaps of another man, perhaps of ten other men—was totally foreign to their ideas of feminine "mental health." Too often in these discussions, the medical mask would slip, and I would find myself facing not the calm professional but the outraged man. The disgusted son, husband, and father would look at me—surely a hoax cleverly disguised as a "nice woman" —with ill-concealed anxiety and dislike. "You are entitled to your subjective opinions, Miss Friday. But have you any medical qualifications to back up your ideas?"

As late as February 1973, the noted "permissive" Dr. Allen Fromme would take a similar position in daring *Cosmopolitan* magazine. "Women do not have sexual fantasies," Dr. Fromme wrote, and went on with patronizing kindness: "How do we know? Ask a woman, and she will usually reply, No. The reason for this is obvious: women haven't been brought up to enjoy sex . . . women are by and large destitute of sexual fantasy."

Needless to say, this reinforced the need to deny the practice of sexual fantasy among the millions of Cosmo Girls who read these words, not only when talking to eminent medicos like Dr. Fromme but even to themselves. *Of course,* most women told Dr. Fromme that they did not have sexual fantasies; no woman wanted to be thought sexually "weird" when faced with what seemed to be expert medical opinion, that if she did, she was totally outside the "normal" experience of her sisters. Dr. Fromme may have thought he was being merely descriptive. In fact, he was being normative. A self-fulfilling prophet.

Yet an example of the almost frightening speed with which the experts can revise their ideas on contemporary sexual dos and don'ts was recently printed in the same magazine in February 1975. When a practicing New York psychoanalyst and *Cosmo*'s own monthly psychiatric-advice columnist could say this:

"... all women have sexual fantasies, though sometimes they won't admit it, even to themselves. Fantasies are make-believe states used to enhance reality. A woman making love to one man may imagine that several other men are watching. ... Her fantasy provides a safe way to explore the erotic possibilities of a situation that might be very threatening or guilt-producing if she acted it out."

The psychoanalyst goes on to say: "A fantasy can give a woman an added sense of life and all its possibilities. It is the *unexamined* corners of the mind that breed neurosis and fear—not the portions of ourselves we know, recognize and accept."

When *My Secret Garden* was published, I was happy to find other doctors coming forward to support my feelings that sexual fantasies were not necessarily a sign of neurosis, but were, instead, a sign of a woman's sexual exuberance and life. Dr. Leonard Cammer, chairman, Section on Psychiatry, Medical Society of the State of New York, endorsed my views, as did the noted founder and executive director of SIECUS. (Sex Information and Education Council of the U.S.), Dr. Mary Calderone. And yet the anxiety that the subject aroused in many medical men would not abate: the validity of my statistical methods was attacked. "But all the women you talked to volunteered to do so," was the way this objection usually ran. "They are a self-selected sample. How can you extrapolate from what these exhibitionistic volunteers tell you? How can you say that their experiences are also shared by their sisters in the silent majority?"

This same argument was used against Kinsey and Masters and Johnson when their research was published, but time has proven that their studies not only voiced the views of the people who volunteered but also spoke

4

for the broad spectrum of Americans in general. In addition, I note no reluctance in the works of psychoanalysts themselves, beginning with Freud, to base their theories of human nature on that tiny fraction of the human race that has laid itself bare on the analytic couch. The vast majority of the human race has never figured in any psychoanalytic survey or clinical documentation of human behavior—and still any psychoanalyst you talk to will unhesitatingly tell you "all" people pass through certain stages of the Oedipus complex. It is my feeling that if over two thousand women from all parts of the country, of all ages, marital status, and economic classes write that they have these or those sexual fantasies that make them feel this way or that, their feelings and experiences are going to be shared by the great majority of all women. "In my practice," says Dr. Sonya Friedman, a Detroit clinical psychologist and marriage counselor, "I am continually struck by how much more we are alike than we are different."

In the end, I must leave the validity of what I am saying to you, the reader, to judge. If this book awakens no resonance in you, if you feel no recognition or empathy between yourself and the women who speak in these pages, it is not that you are odd—it is only that I am wrong about you. But for the rest of my readers, I offer the message that is contained in almost every letter I have received. "Thank God you opened the discussion about women's sexual fantasies. I thought I was the only one who had these ideas. I was afraid to tell my husband [priest, doctor, or whoever]. because I was afraid he would think I was some kind of weird freak. I felt like a pervert, so guilty and alone. . . ." My message is, Welcome. You are not alone.

I believe it is individual anxiety that makes so many people unable to accept the idea of sexual fantasy in others. The portrait of women it evokes is too new, too frightening—above all, too much at war with all our past stereotypes of women as maidens, mothers, "ladies."

People laugh nervously when the subject of *My Secret Garden* and sexual fantasies comes up. Some people turn red and tell me they never read pornography or else they nervously light a cigarette and dismiss the whole subject as "boring." When *Garden* was published, I became depressed by the anxiety/dismissal 'mirth the book aroused in many women and men, friends and strangers. My husband helped me. "Freud was dismissed as a scandal and a dirty old man," Bill said, "because he talked about masturbation and the sexuality of children. Up till then, people thought children were 'pure' as angels. When Freud talked about sex and incestuous desires, he was called a pornographer too." Of course, I am in no way comparing my work or myself to Freud; but I do think we are living through a time in sexual history as emotionally loaded as Freud's own. By trying to understand the secret thoughts of women—the emerging sex—we may succeed in unscrambling the sexual bigotry of the past. Only in this way will we be able to understand the distorted man-woman relationship that has led to the frightening anger between the sexes today. I hope this book will help.

Our real world . . . from the morning paper to the late late television movie . . . is saturated with commercial sex, romantic sex, and, yes, violent sex. These emotions and images stay in our minds—along with all the other desires and drives we are born with. What is a woman to do with all these ideas? One thing she does is shape them closer to her heart's desire, using the sexual stimuli she likes, softening or discarding the images that turned her off, inventing her own sexual fantasies. If these reveries stimulate her sexually while she goes about her daily routine, I'm all for it. If a few lustful and erotic reveries make the housework go by "as if in a dream," why not?

Probably the most important thing to remember about fantasies is that they are not facts, not deeds; they are not "acting out." Summoning up an erotic image in the imagination does not necessarily mean we want to bring it into reality. In fact, very often the fantasy itself discharges the forbidden energy and entirely eschews the need for acting out. In the same way that dreams at night can be said to be psychotic discharges of the mind that allow us to be sane during the day, fantasies of even the most primitive, regressive nature help us to be adult and responsible in our real behavior.

If anyone man or woman, lives out Freud's dictum that a fulfilled life contains both love and work, I don't care what fantasies that person has. If a woman has daydreams of making it with Napoleon's horse, but says she is satisfied with her life, who am I, or who is any doctor, to tell her that she is strange?

Today. for the first time in history, women are encouraging each other to be more sexually free and accepting. As we do, is it surprising that men are now becoming the first line of defense against the breakup of the old morality? It is men who have become wary and critical of women's new role as sexual initiator and free agent. "Love" itself is suddenly raised as the banner under which many men march. "Don't you love me anymore?" suddenly asks the husband who always claimed that his own casual philanderings "have nothing to do with my wife," when he learns that she has been having a little afternoon peccadillo of her own . . . or, yes, a sexual fantasy starring his best friend.

I find men's sexual anxiety today understandable. I am sympathetic to it; women have changed so much in recent years. And men have not. In fact, if you are a woman who is not sympathetic to men today, and you call yourself a "liberated" woman, you should question your insensitivity. Are you happier in your new freedom because it gives you a chance to "get back at men" . . . or because you see it as an opportunity at last to make things better for both of you? Sex never was the simple piece of cake Hugh Hefner sells to men; women's questioning of a sexual status quo that was questionable to begin with must be disquieting if not threatening to men. I'm not saying that a lot of men—the *machos,* for instance—don't deserve their discomfort. But a lot don't. I suppose what it comes down to is that if you're a woman who wants men in your life, you've got to take your responsibility along with your liberation.

The as-yet-unplotted possibilities of women's sexuality, given almost surrealistically vivid form and image in fantasy, not only frightens men but women too. Think of all that desire unleashed, desire he may not be interested in or able to satisfy, appetites mother would never have approved of, sexual *power* she doesn't know what to do with. (How many women know how to make the first move? Should she pick up the telephone, reach for his hand, his cock? Should she say, "Please, I want you to go down on me?" And how many men would reject her if she did? Oral sex may be "intellectually" accepted today, but as you will see from the women in this book—if you have not already discovered it for yourself—there are a great number of men who are unskilled, unpracticed, or unwilling to do what they say.)

We are not yet ready to accept the simple proposition that female sexual power added to male sexual power equals better sex for both. And yet the truth is that the foundation of our myth of male sexual superiority is riddled with deception and fakeroo. Worse, it gives the poor man who believes it an awful superman's burden to carry. *Dominance* and *superiority* are words you use when you go to war, not to bed.

Henry Miller wrote me a letter about *My Secret Garden:* "I've always suspected that women had richer, wilder, fantasies than men. From my limited experience with women I must also add that I have found them more capable of abandoning themselves completely in intercourse than men. In a good healthy sense I would say, to use an old-fashioned word, that they are more 'shameless' than men. . . . Men are only beginning to perceive the true nature of women's being. They have created a false image of her. She is neither an angel nor a bitch in heat. If she is no longer an enigma, she is certainly an everlasting source of wonder and rich in unexplored possibilities in every domain of life."

If I prefer Henry Miller's approach to women's fantasies to that of many psychiatrists, it is because his view of life is large enough to see fantasy as enriching human experience, and not the mark of pathology.

Far from being a perversion of our deepest and most intimate moments together, sexual fantasies answer the need for variety that exists in the best of relationships. To those who think it is a crime to consciously retreat into the secret garden of your mind while in the arms of your beloved, let me quote Dr. Ray Birdwhistle of the University of Pennsylvania. An overly closed idea of marriage, he says, leads to pathology. "Privacy is disallowed as being disloyal. But if the couple wants intimacy, both partners need to refresh themselves with privacy. That implies also being allowed to withdraw without guilt. It is only in the private kingdom of the mind that one can enjoy fantasies. And what held together romantic love in the first place? A rich, lusty, sweet and sad, vengeful and even violent fantasy life" [*New York* magazine, February 1973].

On the last page of *My Secret Garden,* I asked readers to contribute their own sexual fantasies and comments for the book you now hold. It is from the shape these letters took that I have devised the form of this book. Part One deals with the very frequent question of readers, "Where Do Sexual Fantasies Come From?" Part Two, "The Uses of Sexual Fantasy" concerns the role these imaginary, erotic scenarios play in the lives of many women.

As you will see, I have not so much tried to theorize on my own; I have tried instead to organize the material my readers sent in to illustrate the answers to these questions they have raised in their own lives. I believe we live in a time when it is of paramount importance that women learn to speak unashamedly, so that we may learn from each other. I did not ask my readers for all the information they sent me, but I am very grateful that they felt it "right" to try to trace for themselves, and me, the origin of their fantasies and the context in which they appear in their lives.

It is, of course, impossible to analyze any particular woman's fantasy without knowing her, and understanding the full meaning of why she has chosen any particular event or symbol to express her erotic excitement. But that was never my purpose. I began research for *My Secret Garden* in 1968 . . . I began to work on this book in 1973. I wanted to see if the intervening five years had made any significant difference in the attitudes of women toward sexual fantasies. I am pleased to say that while I would characterize the majority of fantasies in *Garden* as various strategies women had devised to handle or disarm sexual guilt, the fantasies I have collected for this book are much more characterized by pleasure and guiltless exuberance. Poets are often called the conscience of a nation; I believe our sexual fantasies are mirrors of the women we would like to become.

I don't think anyone can read the letters in the pages that follow and not be as touched as I was, not only by the feelings expressed but by the outpouring of honesty and the unglossy portrait they give of their lives. What impresses me most is that, although I guaranteed that all contributions would be anonymous, over half the women who wrote signed their full names and gave their addresses—as contrasted to one woman in ten who signed her real name to the letters I collected for *Garden* five years ago.

While I have kept my half of the agreement—all names, professions, geographical, and other too revealing biographical data have been changed—I am moved by the courage of my readers in wanting to speak to me without disguise. As one twenty-five-year-old woman wrote, "I believe that self-acceptance is the first step toward maturity. So that I can believe in myself, I want you to believe in me and what I wrote. And so I am signing my full name." □

PART ONE

WHERE DO
SEXUAL FANTASIES
COME FROM?

CHAPTER ONE

CHILDHOOD

It is evident that fantasies have value in and of themselves to the fantasizers. . . . From the time they were little girls, women have been told "not to think about such things." By bringing women's sexual thoughts into the open the book gives them permission to fantasize and, in so doing, increases the possibility that women thereby also derive permission to experience real life sex more fully, more easily, more rewardingly.

—Dr. Mary Calderone
Review of *My Secret Garden*
SIECUS Report, May 1974

☐ In *My Secret Garden,* there was a chapter called, "Where Did a Nice Girl Like You Get an Idea Like That?" It put forth my feeling that many of our fantasies spring from a time long before the world is ready to acknowledge our sexuality—childhood itself. No great pioneering idea on my part, Freud's work on infantile sexuality dates from the turn of the century. More recently, the eminent authority on childhood psychology, Dr. Arnold Gesell, conducted a study on infant behavior. He placed a fifty-six-week-old boy in front of a mirror, naked. What the child saw of his own body excited him so much that Dr. Gesell was able to photograph him with an erect penis. If a boy barely one year old can have an erotic experience, is it surprising that little girls—usually more precocious than boys—can also be said to be sexual beings almost from birth?

And yet the idea is still unacceptable to most people. Childhood is pictured as a time of ribbons, fairy tales, and lemonade. Adults notoriously forget that they were once children too; they close off their minds to early sexual memories—those embarrassing or shameful events connected perhaps with anxieties about masturbation. I am not suggesting that the sugar and spice of little girls' childhoods are only a false facade. That aspect is real. But so is our sexuality.

So far, I have received over two thousand letters from women who sent me their sexual fantasies in response to the invitation on the last page of *My Secret Garden.* Many were from highly educated women; an equally great number were from people who probably never read Freud. It didn't matter. The cumulative truth of their personal experience confirmed my view that sexual fantasies are often born out of remembered childhood events. These letters cheered me in a very significant way: I loved the self-acceptance they showed, the refusal to continue to carry the age-old feminine burden of shame and guilt. "Let me tell you a bit about myself first," these openhearted letters often begin. The writers want me to *see* them as they are; they want some recognition for the courage with which so many of them lead their lives, even if they ask me not to print their names. "My first sexual experience was when I was about four years old. The little boy who lived next door came over and he . . . etc." No apologies are given, no anatomical details are glossed over or prettified. There is an intuitive understanding that ladylike language would be counterproductive to the purpose we are both striving for . . . that facts are facts and moral judgments are irrelevant. While names, geographical locations, and occupations in these letters have been changed, I have preserved all other biographical details. I feel only out of the richness and density of facts about someone's life can we come to see that she is a woman just like ourselves.

I believe this is important work that women must do together, and I am glad that there are so many willing to lay their lives on the line to help tear down the curtain of silence behind which we have had to hide our erotic selves. It left each woman feeling isolated, an all-too-easy victim to the assumption that only men knew "all about" sex and what "a real woman" was. Behind this barrier, which was marked Innocence, but should more rightly have been named Ignorance, the sexual exploitation of women went on during practically all of recorded history—a time that, thanks to women's new openness and honesty with one another, is coming to an end.

Another significant difference between the letters of 1968 and these new ones is that in *Garden* the average age of the women who contributed was about thirty; they were of the generation born around the time of World War II. The world they grew up in was very different than today's. In that book, the greatest number of fantasies I collected centered around themes of imaginary force and rape, abduction, domination, the anonymous man whom the woman never sees again—all of which are psychological strategies for allowing the woman to have the most thrilling sexual experiences in her fantasies, but all under the slogan, "It wasn't my fault; he made me do it." In other words, *sexual guilt and its avoidance* was the great emotion shared by most women who contributed to *Garden.*

The average age of women who sent in their fantasies for inclusion in this book is about twenty-two. They grew up in the age in which Elvis Presley was bringing a new kind of blatant sexuality to pop music, they entered their own sexual years to the songs of the Beatles. I am not saying that the music of their time directly influenced their approach to life (although often it did), as much as it reflected a whole new era of freedom of sexual expression. The fantasies in this book fill me with admiration for these young women. I am struck by their pride in their sexuality and their pleasure in its exercise—if not in their lives, at least in their fantasies. They are not at all frightened by the sexuality of their earliest years. They aren't into guilt at all.

In memory, there is security. One of the first signs that infants are maturing is the ability to allow mother out of their sight without tears of fear or rage. The baby has begun to believe in the reality of memory—to recognize there is a correspondence between her inner world and the reality "out there." Remembered figures do not vanish into a void, but come back. In time, the baby is freed by this inner certainty and reliance upon memory; she comes to enjoy her periods of solitude. Secure in a base of remembered happiness, the little child can turn her attention forward to learning new things: how to crawl around her crib, perform experiments with her toys and/or body, the pleasures of watching patterns of light cross the ceiling.

So it is in our sexual years. Whenever periods of sexual boredom, anxiety, or frustration come along, we tend to return to childhood scenes of remembered erotic happiness. These will be images or events that happen to the baby that are of an erotic nature. Something is imagined or felt by the little girl, something comes into view that stimulates her. The child does not yet know, nor does she need to know, that these are specifically sexual feelings. She only knows that they make her *feel good* . . . excited, stimulated, flushed with life. Nobody has yet told her she is not to touch herself "down there" . . . that she is not supposed to look at this or think that or do any of the other 999 things that "nice little girls" do not do. She goes over the stimulating incident again and again in memory, almost as a form of sympathetic magic to make the experience recur; it is the same form of primitive logic that made the cavemen draw pictures of deer when they wanted to meet them on the hunt.

This is truly our Age of Innocence. The knowledge of good and evil (conventionally viewed) had not yet been forced upon us. Is it any wonder that we withdraw to these happy memories, these simple joys, during our grown-up times of stress, frustration, or boredom? We were safe and felt alive then; memory allows us again to draw upon these emotions in fantasy.

Unfortunately, it is a period of childhood that does not last long. Very soon the little girl begins to notice that when she says this or does that her parents frown or quickly change the subject. The long series of don'ts are laid on her: the very lack of explanation behind these illogical commands make them more frightening and ominous. She becomes aware that various aspects of her thought or behavior are not to be mentioned. She learns concealment and evasion—but in her mind, at least, *she does not stop having these ideas that make her feel good*. They are too exciting to give up. Guilt and silence turn her memories into fantasies. Again and again, I receive the wildest, most ravenously erotic fantasies from women who begin by writing, "I was very strictly brought up by puritanic parents. . . ."

But while guilt is a heavy load to carry, it is not without innate benefits too; it adds a terrific charge of daring and defiance to sex, of forbidden thrills and excitement to heretofore innocent memories. In the last fantasy that closes this chapter, Joyce writes, "I think that what makes all my sexual activity so enjoyable to me is that my parents were so strict with me when I was growing up." Behind the silence with which she faces the world, the child begins to play over and over again with her taboo ideas, elaborating, adding elements that heighten their erotic charge, changing details with infinite care to ever-increase the orgasmic effect. In our outlawed memories, our first fantasies begin.

Like Joyce, Dorothy too begins her letter by discussing her "strict upbringing." She can remember lying in bed as a child and thinking about her fantasies. "I was never able to banish these deliciously nasty thoughts from my mind," she writes. What heightened her pleasure in these erotic scenarios was to imagine them while she could hear her mother moving around in another part of the house. Right under her mother's nose, so to speak, she could play with these forbidden thoughts. In the secrecy of her mind, she could be sexually defiant.

Carla's letter is not so much the work of an imagination like Dorothy's as it is a collection of resummoned actualities. This loving evocation of the past can be

defined as sexual fantasy too: it is the substitution of
a remembered scene for present reality. "I like to go over
my memories when I have nothing else to do," writes
Carla. "It gives me a warm feeling to remember all the
people in my life, because I liked so many of them."

I have found that this kind of fantasy, which sticks
very close to actual events of the past, is almost always
the mark of someone with low levels of sexual anxiety
and/or guilt. When memories carry too heavy a charge
of psychic pain, the fantasizer usually drops or disguises
them, putting an emotional distance between herself and
the ideas that excite her. She makes up imaginary events,
uses imaginary people to express her eroticism; she can
almost be said to see herself in the third person in her
fantasy scenes—all this incredible sex is not happening
to *me*, it is happening to *her*.

I hasten to add here that this does not mean that
imaginary fantasies are the work of puritanic or guilt-
ridden minds. I would say instead that they are the work
of creative minds that need strategies other than memory
over a distance of time to overcome inhibitions. Dorothy's
fantasies may be more the works of imagination than
Carla's, but nobody reading Dorothy's six scenarios could
feel they were invented by an inhibited woman.

What is most interesting about Carla's letter to me
is that while her memories of past (and present) sexual
experiences would shock or horrify most people, Carla
herself speaks of them all very fondly, with total acceptance of every man, every sexual encounter—with less guilt
about breaking even the incest barrier than most women
would feel about kissing a stranger at a party. She speaks
of her memories with no bravado, no shouts of defiance
that might make us feel she was protesting too much.
"This is how I am," her letter seems to say, "this is what
I do, neither more nor less." It is her life of which she
always speaks, and it does not occur to her for one second
that she does not have every right in the world to do
with it what she will. □

Dorothy

I have just finished reading your book, *My Secret Garden,* and I can truly state that it has changed my life for the better. It took my husband and I four evenings to read it, and those four nights produced the most fantastic sex of our entire married life. I had no idea that knowing about other women's sexual fantasies would turn him on so, and now I think I have the courage to describe some of my own to him, which I've never done before. You see, I had a very strict upbringing. Actually, I suppose it was no more strict than most women's, certainly no worse than that of the other girls I grew up with. But looking back now, I can see it's a miracle that I grew up with any feelings of sexuality whatsoever, given the fact that the atmosphere around our home was that sex just wasn't nice.

Let me say that I'm twenty-six, have been married for a year to a wonderful man I lived with for a year before we married, have no children, and I have a good job as an executive secretary. My husband and I are middle class, both with college educations.

I know now that I have always engaged in sexual fantasy, but up until this point, I felt very guilty and ashamed of my fantasies, and even tried very hard to keep from having them. I can remember how guilty I felt as a little girl when I went to church with my parents, and knew what a terrible little sinner I was for having had those wicked thoughts during the week. I used to pray for salvation (although no one in my family was terribly religious . . . it's just that I was terribly sexual, I suppose). However, I was never able to banish these deliciously nasty thoughts from my mind; lying in bed as a child and thinking about them, even as I heard my mother moving about the house, made them all the more thrilling. Many of my fantasies stem from these early childhood daydreams, and have never lost their impact. Now, your delightful book has finally enabled me to relax with a guilt-free conscience and enjoy them.

21

As I have jotted down the basic themes before starting this letter, I see that I have at least six basic fantasies—each one involves a different position, and I adapt the appropriate fantasy to coincide with the particular position I'm actually in in bed. Below are a couple of my favorites:

1. (I use this one while being manipulated by hand before intercourse.) It's in the 1800s, and I am a beautiful, homeless, penniless young maiden on a voyage by ship to America. The ship's captain (handsome, rugged, much older) has agreed to take me, even though I have no money for my passage. After we are underway, though, I soon realize that there *will* be a payment demanded of me, and I am helpless to resist. (Do I want to be thrown overboard in the middle of the Atlantic?) I am the only woman aboard a ship of rugged, lusty, men, and they all stare at me with desire and longing for my exquisite body. The captain, however, saves me for himself. Since he knows I am a virgin and doesn't want to actually deflower me (I justify this dubious morality of his by making the setting in a very non-permissive time in history), my requirement is to always be by his side, where he can lift my long skirt with one hand and enter me slowly and passionately with his fingers while he is otherwise engaged in commanding his ship. I, of course, am embarrassed and mortified, and I wriggle around as if to get away from his hand, but he only continues with more force and stronger manipulation of my clitoris, until finally I am so excited and turned on (against my will) that I scream out, "Oh fuck me, FUCK ME!" and the whole crew of the ship gathers around to look and comment in amazement at this demure little maiden panting and screaming, with their captain's hand up her dress. At this point, I've usually had an excellent orgasm, and do *indeed* speak those words, to which my hubby happily accommodates, as that is what he has been waiting for. He has no idea what has been going on in my head to bring me to such a frenzy—he only knows his fingers drive me *wild!*

2. (This is for the male-superior position.) I am a schoolteacher in a rural school, and several young, lusty farm boys have cornered me in the one-room schoolhouse after school. Their purpose is a bet: one of the boys (a huge, fair-haired brute with an enormous cock) has bet the others that he can fuck me until I beg for more. They throw me down across my own desk on my back, pull up my dress, pull off my panties, and while the other boys are holding my arms and legs, this big stud goes to work, ramming it in, accompanied by the taunts and encouragements of his friends. (Such as "Shove it in!" "Give it to her!" "Make her scream!") All the time he's saying, "Come, baby, come—cream on me!" while he massages my body with his huge hands. The boys holding my legs spread them wider apart so that he can get deeper into my struggling, writhing body, and he keeps on thrusting away, all the time using his filthiest words, imploring me in a strong but gentle voice to come all over him. I prolong this part as long as it takes me to reach my climax, and it's always a blockbuster. In fact, writing this down seems to bring the whole image flowing back to mind so strongly, I'm really getting turned on. These images had never entered my mind before except during sex.

As I said before, I have a different fantasy for everything including cunnilingus and fellatio, but I'm not going to write them all down or I'd end up writing a book myself. I will say they include such participants as a horse, a dog, Indians, a doctor, and a headmaster in a girl's school. I change roles in each one, and sometimes I'm beautiful and sophisticated, while in others I am childish or simpleminded. Each one is elaborate, but so familiar and dear to me that the right one just pops into my mind without my even consciously willing it. I've truly always thought of these fantasies as my "private little world," and I use them also while masturbating. They make sex more vivid and meaningful for me, and I don't think I could bear to be without them.

As I said before, thanks to your wonderful book, I'm no longer going to try.

I absolutely promise that these fantasies are legitimate, and I'd be glad to write them all down for you if you should want me to, so the name and address are legit also. I look eagerly forward to your next book, and I do hope I may have been of some small help—you've helped me more than I can tell you.

Carla and Tom

Since my brother and I read your book, *My Secret Garden*, we have felt great relief to know we were not the only brother and sister who fuck. May we add our bit to your next book? I hope it will help others like us. Tom and I don't consider what we're doing "unnatural" at all. Being in bed with him seems like the most natural thing of all.

I like to go over my memories when I have nothing else to do. It gives me a warm feeling to remember all the people in my life, because I liked so many of them. I remember when I was six that my mother used to scold me when she caught me playing with my cunt, but I always had the desire to expose myself to the little boys who came over to play in our yard. I would take off my panties, and I remember several times the older boys would take me into a corner and play with my cunt. Some boys took all their clothes off one day and laid me down on their shirts and pants and worked their fingers up me. I liked it, but it made me sore. I didn't say anything to my mother, because she would stop the boys from coming over to play at our house. The first time a bigger boy took me into the back seat of a car in a garage, he removed all my clothes and spread my legs so far apart I thought he would split me apart. He kept getting closer and closer, and I thought he was examining me. I like the idea that he wanted to see my cunt so closely, but he suddenly proved my reading of what he was up to

24

wrong: he got his mouth into my cunt and was darting his tongue in and out like a snake. I loved it so much that when he wanted to stop I begged him to do it some more. He promised to come over often and do this to me. We found places like our attic, garage, or sheds in the woods. I was very sad the day his family moved to another part of the state, but before he left, he taught me a nice game. He used a weiner to jack me off with and then told me to eat the weiner so that nobody would ever discover I had a weiner in my bedroom. When he moved away, I used to do this and think of him.

When I was old enough to go to school, the boys soon found out that they could get to play with my cunt any time at all. My uncle found the same to be true one summer we spent July and August on his ranch in New Mexico. I have very happy memories of the way my uncle loved to play with my cunt and took me with him when he was making trips around the place. Uncle was very kind to me, and when he sucked my cunt, he did it very gently. I remember one time we were a long way from home, and he found a spot where it was really quiet. He had me undress completely, and he spread out a large quilt, laid me down, and put his tongue in my cunt. At this time, I was nine years old. We had fun, and then he undressed and showed me his cock. I had never seen a grown man's cock before, and I did not understand how it could be so big. He got on top of me and told me to be easy in my mind; he was just going to put the head of his cock up to my cunt. I asked him what would happen then, and he said that he would just do with his cock the way he had always done with his finger, so I wasn't frightened. Instead, did that ever start my desire to have that cock in my cunt. He spread my cunt lips open and gently shoved his cock part way in. His actions just drove me to want that big cock all the way in, just as I had gotten used to shoving a big, rubber, imitation weiner all the way in when I wanted to jack off. (The rubber one was bigger and better than the real ones I had started with.) When my uncle shoved his whole cock in, he found it was easier to do than he had thought. He asked me if I had ever fucked before. I told him about the big rubber weiner. He asked if I had brought it along. I had, and told him how I used it when I was by myself. That made him so excited that after our first fuck he spent two more hours just sucking my cunt. Then he asked me to take his cock in my mouth. I was so afraid that if I said no he would never fuck me anymore that I took his cock and sucked him. He kept telling me to suck harder, and after I had sucked awhile my tongue got sore, so we stopped. When we returned to the house everyone had gone to see a movie, so that left us alone. I was so tired that I just fell asleep. When I woke up, my uncle was sucking my cunt.

The next day my uncle and aunty had to go into town for a meeting, leaving my brother and I alone. We spent the time looking around because being on a ranch was so new to us. We came across two dogs who were trying to fuck. We watched and it got me so passionate that I stepped backward, up against the front of my brother's pants. He was feeling the same way, because without a word, he put his hands up under my halter, exposing my little breasts and cupping my tits in his hands. We soon were kissing, and he had me walk around to the back of the milk house. When we were there, he pulled my bikinis off and the halter of my sunsuit. We played a bit there that way, and then we made a dash for the house—me running naked all the way—and went to his bedroom. It started that way, just as easy as that, and from then on we have been fucking each other all along very happily and that was twelve years ago. Do you know any other marriages that have continued happily for twelve years? I don't. I wish people who read this letter and feel bad about us would remember that before they criticize. We now live together, and every one of our friends think we are husband and wife. He is very considerate. Unlike most husbands, he shaves every day so that he will not irritate my skin, etc.

One of the letters in *My Secret Garden* spoke about

dogs. When Tom and I read this, we decided to see what it was like. My brother and I started to fuck to get the dog excited. It sure did—he got in between our legs and licked both Tom and me while we were fucking. What a pleasure! When we finished, Tom let his cock go off in me. (I'm on the pill) Tanzy licked my cunt, and Tom just lay back and watched. We let Tanzy lick as long as he wanted, and then he began to get up on his hind legs and hug my leg. That told us he wanted to fuck. Tom had me get up on my knees and he helped Tanzy get his cock in my cunt. We did not know how much cock a dog has, but I soon found out. When he got that knob in my cunt, he had over eight inches of cock shoved up me. Fuck, you never know what it can do to a girl until she gets fucked by her dog. That pink fleshy cock is in my cunt whenever Tanzy has a desire to fuck me. Tom likes to watch his cock plunge in and out of my cunt. One day Tom asked me how it made me feel, and when I told him, we tried to get Tanzy to shove it up Tom's asshole so he could feel what I was feeling. But the hole was too small for Tanzy to get in. Sometimes I get up on top of Tom, and we both lay that way, both our legs apart, bellies up, and Tom lets Tanzy fuck me when we are in this position. Tom's cock rides in the crack of my ass below, and Tanzy is giving it to me from straight above. If I am alone and Tanzy wants to fuck, I place the davenport cushions on the floor and lay on my back. Tanzy is very smart and knows how to fuck me both from the rear and front. I love to fuck him from the front, because I can look down and see his cock entering my cunt, that pink shaft just going in and out. He always licks my cunt clean after we get through fucking.

It was Tom's idea that I write this letter to you, but when I got started typing, I got so excited that he had to help me finish it. My last thought is that anything you fuck that makes you feel good is okay.

□ Jennie is only seventeen, and her childhood isn't that distant. She remembers it very clearly: "Where I was brought up," she says, "sex was pretty much taboo." She is enough a child of our time to say in one breath, "I always consider myself a girl of high morals and always thought I would be a virgin until I was married" . . . and then she goes on to describe her sexual experiences with her boyfriend, whom she plans to marry "in three years."

What I like about Jennie is that she does not feel these contradictions are important enough to comment upon; no apologies or explanations are felt necessary. She is a girl who accepts her own sexuality in her own time; she believes more in her own feelings than the amorphous "rules" in the air. When she says she has no guilt about her sexuality or her fantasies, I believe her.

Jennie's mother clearly grew up in a totally different sexual atmosphere, and although her daughter was aware of this difference between herself and her mother, even as a child of nine, she did not blindly accept her mother's sexual authority: she felt and believed in her own sexuality even more.

Jennie may not be typical of her generation, but there are countless young women like her; the very fact that she wrote me—and with such eagerness—indicated her interest in sex. What I find more significant is the ease, acceptance, and utter naturalness with which she treats that interest. □

Jennie

I have just finished reading your book, *My Secret Garden*. Throughout the book, I kept thinking what it would be like to actually write to you. When I saw your address in the back, I knew I had to write.

First, I'll give you some background information about myself. I am seventeen, and my boyfriend is sixteen. We are both seniors in high school, and plan to get married in three years. I always considered myself a girl of high morals and always thought I would be a virgin until I was married.

Where I was brought up, sex was pretty much taboo. No one ever spoke about it, so I never knew anything about sex. I know that when I was about nine years old I used to get sensual feelings, although at the time I didn't know what they were. I used to take my clothes off and rub my small breasts and my cunt against the cold washing machine, and this made me feel very good. At other times, I would take all my clothes off and run around in the woods across the street. Sometimes my girl friend would come with me, and we would sit and masturbate ourselves or each other. Just thinking about doing these things when I was a kid would get me excited, and the next thing I knew I was doing them or thinking up something new that would make me feel good. Given the puritanic background where I grew up, it's amazing I didn't feel really guilty as a kid, but I didn't. I just knew it couldn't be bad if it felt that good.

Nowadays, I fantasize whenever I have time on my hands . . . or my hands on myself. I don't think I masturbate any more than the average girl, but I don't know much about the average girl. It's a sexy world, so I have sexy thoughts quite a bit. I don't usually fantasize when I have sex with my boyfriend. All I need to hear is his heavy breathing and I get horny. My boyfriend loves to experiment with sex. Sometimes we fuck with him coming in from the back, sometimes sitting up; we even tried it in the shower once.

He likes it when I use my mouth on him. Often, in public, I can't refrain from touching him up. Up until recently, I would never allow him to perform cunnilingus on me, but now I love to feel him sucking my clitoris and slipping his tongue in and out of me.

When I'm by myself masturbating or daydreaming, my fantasies change all the time. My favorite fantasies include being fucked by a lion, a black man, or a cousin

29

of mine. I've always dreamed about trying incest, but I have no brothers. The closest I can get is my cousin. He is ten years older than me. Recently, my grandfather died, and my cousin came up from Georgia for the funeral. We have always been attracted to one another, and during the middle of the night, he came down to where I was sleeping on the sofa. We smoked a jay, and he kissed me. Then we got into some petting. After a while, I told him to go away. Since then, how many times I've wished I hadn't! My chance will come again, but I know I won't let anything happen, because I am very faithful to my boyfriend, and I know he would never have an affair with another girl. But I love to use this story of what happened that night with my cousin as my fantasy; I try all sorts of different endings to it, thinking about all the things that could have gone on between us.

I have no guilt feelings about fantasizing. I love to hear my boyfriend tell me he's going to "fuck me" during intercourse. It really turns me on. Some of my fantasies I share with him. There is one we plan to carry out soon. I told him I wanted him to force himself upon me, to rape me when I said "No" to him. He wants me to fight him off while he tells me he's going to fuck me.

We have not got into "the group thing." It doesn't appeal to either of us. My boyfriend says he doesn't fantasize. Maybe someday he will. I have found that when I do fantasize during sex, it adds to both of our excitement.

Thank you for letting me get this off my chest. I hope it is of some value to you in your studies. Good luck.

☐ One of the pleasures in reading novels or going to the movies is the feeling they give us of how other people live. They seem to enlarge the possibilities of our own lives. Sexual fantasy, too, will often serve the same function, but instead of reading about other people, by an act of emotional imagination, we put ourselves in their shoes and bodies, feel what they feel, experience their sexual joys as if they were our own. In Sarah's fantasies, which follow, I find the one about the male guardian the most interesting. It is evidently born out of childhood experiences—the emotions seem to be of such an early stage of development that even the sexual lines are blurred: Sarah tells us that she plays all roles, both male and female. This is not uncommon in fantasy. We all wonder how other people *are* sexually; in our erotic reveries, we can rehearse their emotions within ourselves. Another signal, I feel, that this fantasy is an imaginative recreation of very early scenes is that Sarah does not really put herself into any of the roles, not even that of "the girl." It all speaks of a time when she was so young that she could not choose to act, but was acted upon. It is not, "I did this or that . . ." but "The girl is told to take a bath . . ." and so on. □

Sarah

My fantasies have some points in common with those in your book, which I loved, and others somewhat different. One of them is recalling some good times with my ex-husband. He would get me pretty excited with foreplay, and then he would put it in, he would make just two or three thrusts, and then he'd sort of back off with just the tip of it in and tease me—"Do you want it, baby? Then you'll have to come and get it! Bring it up to me, baby, climb my pole!" and I would have to raise my hips up and down, and sometimes he would move around a little and pretend he was going to take it out and quit, and I would twist and turn and raise and lower my hips frantically to keep it in and keep the motion going—and of course I'd get hotter and sweatier—doing all the work. And I had really great orgasms that way. I could get on top, but it never worked with me that way—only when I was underneath, and really working at it. (I know some men don't like that at all.)

One other fantasy I have is about a lover I had who

used to have me sit on top of his refrigerator and sort of slide down one rounded corner of it till his tongue was even with my cunt, and he'd stand there with his hands sort of cupping my buttocks to keep me from falling quite helplessly onto the floor, and lap it up like an ice cream cone. Then he'd have me slide down off the refrigerator right onto his big cock—nothing I could do about that either—and waltz me into the bedroom with my toes just off the floor. Our favorite joke was, "Do you want to come over and defrost my refrigerator tonight?"

So much for recalling reality—now for fantasies that are just fantasies. There's one about the little girl who has a male guardian—father or uncle, I never really figured it out. One day, the girl has a little boyfriend come over to play after school and invites him to stay for dinner. The guardian agrees, and the boy telephones home for permission. but is told his parents are going out for dinner, and he has to stay where he is till nine-thirty. if that's not too late. (I play all three roles in this, alternating.) The guardian again says okay. But after dinner, he tells the girl she must go and take her bath, which she does. Then he calls to her and says just to come out in her bathrobe. She does, and then he says to her, "Did you wash your roses good?" She says she did, and he says, "Come lie down over here on the sofa, and let's see if you did." She says no, she doesn't want to show Toby (her little boyfriend) her roses. At this, the guardian gets angry and takes down a little paddle off the mantelpiece and says. "So you don't want to show him your roses, do you? Well, we'll just show him your little bare bottom then," and he takes her over his knee, pulls up her bathrobe. and proceeds to give her a good paddling, turning both of her cheeks pink. Then he stops and says, "Do you want to show Toby your roses?" And she says, "Yes, yes, yes!" So he puts her on the sofa on her back and brings the lamp over, so it can shine very bright, and pushes up a stool for Toby. "Sit there," he commands Toby. Then he opens the girl's legs and examines her minutely, opening the labia around the vagina and the clitoris. Then he scolds the girl, who has stopped crying by now. "You didn't wash very good. We'll have to do better than that." He tells Toby to put his finger in her vagina and hold her open with his other hand while he goes and gets the washrag from the bathroom. Toby is afraid not to do as he is told and gets more and more interested in the process and asks the girl if his finger hurts her, and she says no, it feels good, but will he move his other hand a little, which he does. The guardian comes back with a washrag that he has surreptitiously wet with the raspberry-tasting mouthwash, and telling Toby to keep his finger where it is, he sponges the clitoris and labia—which turn pink from the mouthwash color and the heat its slight antiseptic content generate. The girl tries to twist and turn and says the water's too hot, "It's hot, it hurts! Oh, Toby, kiss it and make it stop hurting." And Toby bends his head and kisses her. By now in this fantasy, I would have come about twice. Sometimes the guardian spanks Toby after this.

By now, I haven't got enough energy left to tell you many details about my daughter's slumber party she had when she was in junior high. The buzzing would kind of quiet down, and I'd think finally I could get to sleep. Then I'd hear a "Whap!" and little moans and giggles. Since then I've imagined planting a tape recorder at one of those parties. Wouldn't it be fun to hear what games they really play and who gets whapped and why?

☐ In the letters that follow, very early experiences are brought to mind. While Claudia is clearly a very healthy and erotic young woman, I like the way she gives herself permission not to hurry into sexual experience before she is emotionally ready for it. "I'm only fourteen years old, so I haven't screwed yet," she says, adding, "but I do enjoy some sex with my boyfriends." Reading her letter, we get the feeling that when she is ready for a full sexual experience, she will do it confidently, easily, and well. She will probably be the one who decides exactly when, where, and with whom it will take place.

The progress of Claudia's life toward full womanly eroticism seems clear; the four next letters help us chart some of the pitfalls that seem to have lain in the way for other women. The difficult terrain is very clearly mapped in Janice's letter. "I deeply love my husband," she writes "(we have been married sixteen years), but I have always been profoundly thrilled by my fantasies, which go back to an episode in my adolescence. . . . To me, now that I dare think about it after reading your book, it seems only natural that women should be aroused by incidents involving urination, given the fact that our sexual parts are so close to our urinary parts."

While the incident that Janice refers to in her fantasy happened during her adolescence, her erotic interest in, and confusion of, urinary and sexual processes most likely began far earlier in her life. By the time "Aunt Bessie" came along, Janice had long since been unconsciously prepared to find the older woman's invitation enough to "drive me out of my mind." Denise's letter, too, reminds us that about the time mother began our toilet-training, she also began telling us not to play with ourselves "down there." It is often a time of tension between mother and daughter—perhaps the first of their lifelong battles. All interest is focused on this one part of the body during this period, the mysteries of sex and urination become interwined—because both seem to be forbidden. Eroticism and excretion become emotionally combined—the vagina is experienced as the seat of a double kind of excitement.

The woman Frank writes about is fascinated by anal play—she calls herself an "anal-erotic." I include his letter not so much for what he tells us about himself, but because his lover is such a clear example of Freud's dictum that the anal stage of development precedes the genital. Frank's lover chooses to live out with him those fantasies that are the outgrowth and expression of early toilet-training experiences . . . as also seems true of Lana, whose fantasy follows Frank's letter. Robyn daydreams happily about the guiltless pleasure of her fiancé giving her an enema. In these letters, I am struck by the marvels of human nature, its recuperative power and above all, its overriding drive for health and self-acceptance. Janice, Denise, Frank's lover, Lana, and Robyn have all taken what might seem at first glance to be behavioral hangups, but I have found in them sources of erotic pleasure instead. I applaud them all. □

Claudia

I have just finished reading your book. Thank you, for it really opened my eyes to the way many women think. Some parts shocked me, other parts disgusted me, but most of it excited me. And I truly believe there are women who feel excited even by the things that turn me off . . . and that's okay for them. I find it exciting that we women are all so different.

I have never been ashamed of my fantasies, but I just didn't know that's what they were. I'm only fourteen years old, so I haven't screwed yet, but I do enjoy some sex with my boyfriends. I have had fantasies ever since I can remember. As a little kid, I imagined I was a harem girl, or a slave girl on sale at a public marketplace. I was always well-developed in the fantasy, although I was actually flat as a board then and didn't have a single pubic hair. In my fantasy, men would walk by me and examine me, but only with their eyes. It wasn't until I was eleven years old that I even began to think and fantasize of guys putting their fingers up me. When I was ten, I stopped being the submissive one in my thoughts, and became the seducer. At night, I would (and still do) think of a foxy guy I know or a handsome teacher and imagine me telling him to suck my tits, while I softly play with his cock.

I "cock watch," naturally. I can't help it. To me, it's just like guys looking at boobs. I sometimes wear sexy clothes, and it excites me to know that I have caused a guy to get a boner. I then imagine what his cock looks like, how large his balls are, how erect it (the dick) is, if he's circumcised or not, etc. You know, all the things girls who like guys enjoy thinking about.

I hope you can use this in your next book. It has excited me just to write about it, because I have never told anyone about these things, except when I was a kid. Thank you again for your book! I think I got my first orgasm while reading it and masturbating myself, but I'm not sure. Thanks anyhow, because it felt good!

Janice

I am so pleased your book opened up an area of discussion which so directly affects my sexual life. Until reading other women's fantasies of urination—the sexual pleasure derived from such ideas—I had felt myself to be "unusual" or worse. I deeply love my husband (we have been married sixteen years), but I have always been profoundly thrilled by my fantasies, which go back to an episode in my adolescence. I have thought about this incident so often, and embroidered on it, that I am no longer quite sure what actually did happen and just what I have added to increase the pleasure thinking about it gives me.

To me, now that I dare think about it after reading your book, it seems only natural that women should be aroused by incidents involving urination, given the fact that our sexual parts are so close to our urinary parts. I sometimes think that if I dared think about many of the things that frighten me, the fear would be replaced so easily by self-acceptance; all that keeps me, and others, from thinking of these fearsome things is the thought that it is sinful to consider them; and yet what can be sinful in just thinking about something?

Here is my fantasy:

I am visiting at the home of an older friend, someone

I call Aunt Bessie, although we are not related. One rainy day, during the visit, as luncheon time approaches, Aunt Bessie and I have two large martinis. Afterward, we sit down at the dining table to eat. Lunch starts with a delicious thin soup, of which I have two servings. Soup is followed by cold cuts, accompanied by steins of cold, foaming beer. For dessert, there are crackers and cheese, with refills of the steins to wash it down. About half an hour after lunch, I get up from my chair and start to leave the room. Aunt Bessie asks where I am going, and I reply: "Sorry, but I have to pee." To this, Aunt Bessie says, "Nonsense, you just think you have to go. Come back here and sit down, and we will split a bottle of champagne." Although I have some doubts as to my ability to retain any longer, all the liquid I have imbibed nevertheless I comply. At this point, I begin to suspect that Aunt Bessie has something "up her sleeve," but just what, I cannot imagine. We sit for a while, drinking the champagne and smoking two or three cigarettes, me feeling more and more uncomfortable by the minute. As I finish the last drop in my glass, I say to Aunt Bessie: "I really must go now, I can't hold it any longer." Aunt Bessie replies: "Well, if you must, you must, but I hope you don't mind if I go with you." Upon arriving in the bathroom, Aunt Bessie asks me to remove my dress and panties and then sit on the toilet seat, but without dropping even a tear for a few moments. Aunt Bessie then kneels down on a cushion placed conveniently to one side of the toilet seat, reaches across my nearest thigh, and proceeds to manipulate my clitoris. As soon as I feel my friend's fingers playing with my clitoris, the desire to void my urine recedes. Aunt Bessie tells me: "Wait until the exact moment of the climax I am going to bring you to, and then let the freshet flow. I guarantee you will have the most ecstatic orgasm any woman can have in this world—or the next, for that matter."

Sure enough, just as Aunt Bessie's skillful fingers bring

37

me up to and push me over the edge, I let my piss come in a rush. It is like coming in two places at once, and the hot piss flowing down my slit and over the pulsating mouth of my vagina nearly drives me out of my mind.

Denise

Thanks for doing *My Secret Garden*—one of the fantasies electrified me, naturally: I saw myself in it. On p. 179, "Faith" calls herself a "urologenic." Obviously, there must be a lot of us if someone put such a fancy label on us! What I want to know is where I can find out more about us—also, I'd surely like to trade fantasies with another like-minded gal—if at all possible. I'd like you to forward my letter to Faith; if you can't do that, it's okay, and I understand. Now maybe you'd like a fantasy along these lines for your next book. I'm gay, by the by, and ecstatically happy about it. Before I understood my fascination with urination, I used to try to turn my fantasies toward intercourse and ejaculation—I thought I had urination mixed up with ejaculation, but I realize it's just not true. It's the accidents people have, especially men or boys, that fascinate me.

My favorite fantasy takes place in a grammar school classroom. Billy, a cute fifteen-year-old, raises his hand to be excused to the bathroom. The teacher carelessly ignores him, then puts him off with repeated "in-a-minutes." At this point in the fantasy, many variations work. A typical version now is that he feels such pressure that he jams his knees together and scoots forward at his desk, trying to "hold it." It doesn't help, and with his face burning, he finds it necessary to let go just a little, every few minutes, to ease the pressure. Soon, the other kids notice, pointing and whispering at the growing puddle under his desk. Billy always wears tight Levi's and has a very cute behind. Sometimes he is made to stand in the corner at the front of the room, where he wets himself in front of everybody.

I only wish I had a notion of how to look for information on this "aberration." Thanks a lot!

Frank

I'm a heterosexual male, and it would seem absurd for me to comment on the sexual fantasies of women. In fact, I'm not even interested in them to any extent; I ran across your *My Secret Garden* by accident and only thumbed through it idly. However, I see you are collecting material, and I have a sort of case history to give to you for what it's worth. This is a lived-out fantasy in which I participated, and frankly, I'm a bit troubled about it in retrospect. It's rather extreme, or so it seems to me, and I wonder if I have encouraged the woman in what may become a harmful sexual aberration.

First, let me set the stage and describe the characters briefly. I'm a middle-aged business executive and quite an ordinary fellow, nothing special about me at all. The woman is nearing forty, a rather intense emotional type but distinctly attractive, married to a man she likes but who is totally impotent due to illness. She is torn between resolve to remain at least technically faithful to her husband and an urgent need for sexual release. I like her, and am sympathetic to her in her problem. The two of us compromised in a pretend affair limited to cunnilingus and fellatio.

But this wasn't wholly satisfactory to either of us. For my part, I enjoy this with an attractive woman, but mostly as only a part of loveplay rather than as an end in itself. She felt guilt-ridden and had difficulty achieving orgasm that way. It just wasn't very good. Until we discovered something else, by a quite accidental move on my part. I was caressing her vulva with my hand preparatory to cunnilingus, when I inadvertently let a finger stray into the crevice of her buttocks, and its tip pressed into her anus. She stiffened and cried out, and almost instantly went into orgasm.

39

Here at last we come to the fantasy itself. She was, in fantasy, an anal erotic. Later, she confessed this to me. She dreamed of having a man thrust his finger through the sphincter of her anus and on up into her rectum. Going further, she imagined his mouth on her there. And, in return, of putting her mouth on him.

Later, we actually did this. I was personally a bit doubtful, to tell the truth. There have been other women in my experience who liked anal loveplay, and I am not particularly averse to it. When I'm in the proper mood, an attractive woman's anus can be exciting as a part of the whole of her. I like everything about women, and although I have never done actual anal intercourse, I often do caress a woman there during loveplay or cunnilingus if she seems to want it. But it turned out that, once released from inhibition, this woman was really avid about this. It was not only the best but almost the only way she could achieve complete orgasm. And for the ultimate experience, she wanted it to be shared. So it became our regular custom to do it to one another. Lying head to toe, I would fasten my mouth over her anus while stroking her vulva and clitoris with the fingers of a hand. She would tuck my penis down between her breasts, hold my testicles aside with one hand, and suck with lips and tongue at my anus.

The actual living out of this fantasy of hers seems to give her a supreme experience. She goes quite mad in her ecstasy. Her anus works in and out against my lips, her vulva positively gushes fluid, she bites and sucks at my anus and crushes my penis between her breasts, her climax when it comes is violent and interminable.

All this is most enjoyable for me too, I'll admit. I'm something of a voyeur, I like to look at an attractive woman in all her intimate places, to see her vulva open pink and wet, her clitoris swell, her little peeplace gape open at the touch of my tongue, her vagina reveal its inner flesh to me, her anus stretch and pulsate as I touch her there. I like to feel her, and smell her, and taste her. And God knows it's a fantastic titillating sensation to have a woman's lips and tongue sucking and probing at me, to have her breasts caress my penis until it spurts over them and her belly.

But all this, good though it is, somehow pales in comparison to the real thing for me. I like giving her pleasure in this way; I enjoy it myself. But it's all only play to me; I remain unaffected in the ultimate sense. But for her, it seems to be rapidly assuming the proportions of an obsession. She doesn't want it any other way now. I'm worried—she's really a very nice person, and I do like her—lest I may be encouraging her in a sexual aberration that may eventually do her harm.

Oh, well, you've listened long enough. I don't expect you to reply, and perhaps this report may be of no use to you at all. But if you're interested in the sexual fantasies of women, here's one that came to life. You're welcome to use all or any part of this account as you like, no obligation. In any case, good luck to you in writing more about this interesting subject of women and their fantasies.

Lana

Congratulations on a sensitive piece which rightfully credits women with a high degree of creativity.

After reading your book, it sounded like fun to write down a fantasy I have been having—it seems a little more difficult to share it. Actually, my fantasy does not materialize during sex, but rather acts as kind of a "sleeping pill" when I have had a particularly tiring day at work.

It begins as I am sitting in a waiting room which is painfully antiseptic and severe. I feel very uncomfortable being there. for it seems it is somewhat against my will. Other girls are seated around me also nervously shifting in their chairs.

Finally. my name is called by a woman who resembles an old grade-school librarian. Very unchic and clinical. She shows me into a huge office painted white, with a cold metal examination table in the middle. She asks that I remove my clothes and carry them to the corner of the room. When I bend down to put them there, she tells me to stay in that position while she prepares an injection to tranquilize me. She finally returns and feels all over me for the correct site—usually on my rear. As she is giving me the shot, three men enter the room. One is deadly serious, and the others are his students. They are all surprised at the position I am in. The teacher appears cross with the woman for not doing a better job of relaxing me.

I am told to mount the examination table. I do and lie on my back. But one of the students laughs and asks me to turn over, saying he needs the relaxed end up. It is at that point, out of the corner of my eye, with my head resting on my hands, that I see a large machine being wheeled in with a tubular device attached to a long rubber hose. One of the students asks me to relax and spread my legs as far as they will go, while the other student, amid sideways winks and donning rubber gloves, lubricates my rectum with his fingers. The teacher then slowly and with some difficulty (because I keep tightening my muscles) inserts the tube into my rear and announces that this is an enema designed with both an outflow and inflow suction.

Water swishes, legs are held apart, and I am constantly told to relax. After a while, it is all over, and the tube is removed. By then I am usually asleep.

Should I need to fantasize further, I am prepared.

The teacher tells me I am to be the model for a mold or casting of a dildo to better fit all women. Another injection, and then I am turned over. My legs are spread on a trapeze affair suspended from the ceiling. The students busy themselves with a thorough douching of my vagina, while the teacher feels my breasts and asks me if it hurts.

Then another machine is wheeled in with a larger tube inserted into that clean vagina. The plaster oozes out of the tube and seems to fill my whole body. It's warm and keeps expanding. One of the students pushes his hand on my stomach, while the other closes the slit with his fingers. Meanwhile, the doctor inserts a lubricated thermometer in my rectum.

Others are called to help remove the casting—usually men that I have never had affairs with, but have thought about it. They enter the room slightly surprised to see me, but don rubber gloves and aid in taking out the form.

The final bliss comes when it is tried out on the librarian-type.

I am amazed that I wrote this, but really did have fun doing it. It is a genuine fantasy.

Robyn

I just finished reading your book, *My Secret Garden*, and I must admit I enjoyed it very much.

To give you a bit of my background, I'm female, eighteen. and am presently engaged to be married in one and a half years. Please, no comments! I've had enough objections from my parents and relatives already! John and I are very much in love, although we've known each other only eight short months!

I've had sex with two other guys before John, but I never really enjoyed it. With John, every minute we are making love is heaven. I am the first girl John has ever fucked. and John is the only guy who's made me reach a climax. We fuck about three or four times a week (I'm on the pill). usually in his car, occasionally we rent a motel room, although I have to be home by 1:30 A.M. I guess I should tell you our favorite ways of fucking before I tell you my fantasies. First of all, we both get greatest satisfaction with me on top. He can touch my clitoris when I'm this way, and I can fondle his balls. When in the car, I kneel over him while he's sitting. and this way he can use one finger on my clitoris, and another finger up my anus. I adore the feeling I get when his finger is in my asshole. I come the best this way. We use every possible word, while fucking. I love to hear him say what he's doing, and really letting the words flow. However, we never use these words *any other* time. I also enjoy a good sound spanking on my bare bottom before making love. (He can't stand me spanking him, though.) It feels great when he puts a lotion on my fiery bottom afterward.

We both enjoy the sixty-nine position, with me on top. This way he can also use his hand. I can't come when he's not using a finger on my clitoris. Often, he'll go down on me before we make love; I usually come while he's doing this.

Now, for fantasies. I guess mine are basic, not too unusual. I often daydream of having sex with another woman, but I never think of this while we're fucking. I'd really like to try it with a girl, but truthfully, I don't know anyone I could do it with. By the way, none of my girl friends, except one, know that John and I fuck. If the opportunity ever arose, I'd definitely try it. (And I'd *never* tell John.)

I'd also like to pretend that John was a doctor, and he'd have to give me an enema. I can see him wearing the kind of white gauze mask that doctors wear and leaning over me. I am on a special gynecological table, with my feet in the stirrups, but because he is going to carefully examine my anus before giving me an enema, I am lying facedown, so I am all spread open for him, my cunt and my anus. First, he pokes his finger in my asshole and tries to look in. But he can't see enough. So he takes out a kind of surgical pliers and warms the cold metal in a bowl of warm water. Then he inserts the pliers in my anus, and when they are in good and deep, he slowly opens them so he can have a good look in. For some reason of anatomy I don't understand, he has to put his fingers in my vagina while he is examining my asshole. Perhaps this helps open it up more. Then when he has it figured out, he says to me, "Well, I will have to give you an enema. That will fix you up." But instead of having me sit on a toilet, he puts me in a kind of swing, so that I am supported under the shoulders, and from the knees down, but my bottom is hanging naked down below. John brings in an enormous enema bottle and hangs it up high over my head. "This will really fix you up," he says, and begins to insert the rubber pipe into me. He is down below the canvas swing, so I can't really see him, but he's shoving in inches and feet of rubber piping, really shoving it in. And then as he turns on the warm water, he leans over to kiss me. As he does so, he puts his fingers on my clitoris and lovingly plays with it. I can feel the water gently running up through me; John is holding my cunt lips tenderly in his hands and telling me I'll be all right soon. The feeling is very peaceful, but even as I write this, I can feel myself almost beginning to come.

That fantasy may seem a bit gross, but I'd really like it to happen. (Wherever could I get stirrups and the canvas swing and such?) I don't know if I'll ever get enough nerve to ask John to do this, but maybe if I get drunk enough . . . I'm sure he would agree—he never refused to try anything. I'd also like to shave all my pubic hair off, but he is repulsed by the idea.

We also masturbate together (I seldom do it alone), and we've seen each other pee. It's most romantic in the dark deep woods!

I hope I've helped you in some way. Please hurry and publish your next book. I can hardly wait to read it.

Maybe, I'll invite you to our wedding! Remember—SEX IS BEAUTIFUL!

P.S. He also loves to suck on my large tits. He can't wait till I'm pregnant.

P.P.S. I also get turned on by hard porno. (He doesn't.)

☐ In all the fantasies that follow in this chapter, the writers themselves describe their fantasies as growing out of childhood experiences—or else their early beginnings are evident in the emotions they express. I always feel grateful to women like Ivy and Sophie who write to confirm the value of sexual fantasies in their lives; just as their own therapists have told them that sexual fantasies do not mean they are freaks, so have several other psychoanalysts written to me of the usefulness to human health and happiness of sexual fantasy. As part of their therapeutic approach, these doctors have begun to encourage their more inhibited patients to invent their own fantasies, often beginning by having them read *My Secret Garden* first.

I especially appreciate the generosity of Dr. Harrison's letter, not just toward me but clearly toward all his women patients. The fact that he would also enclose his own fantasy makes him even more dimensional to me, not just a doctor but a man too. We may not all be able to afford, or want, psychotherapy, but the experiences these women have shared with us—acknowledging how difficult it was for them to accept and enjoy the guilt-ridden early sexual pleasures of childhood—can help us all. You were sexual as a child; the thrills and sensations you felt then are still with you. You may have felt guilty about it when you were six or ten, but you are grown-up now and can understand how unnecessary this guilt is. More important, you can put those early sexual experiences and emotions to work for you. When we were children, many of us were made to memorize a passage from the Bible: "When I was a child, I spake as a child. . . . When I became a man, I put away childish things." I submit that this is not entirely correct. We may put away childish words and games, but our earliest sexuality is the foundation on which our sexual maturity grows. These women recognize this. Maybe you can learn from them. ☐

Ivy

I've just finished reading *My Secret Garden*. For me, it was one of many approaches I am currently taking to work through numerous sexual hang-ups. Mostly it helps by confirming my therapist's statements that my fantasies and sexual desires are normal, shared by many others.

I am thirty-one, married nine years, two children, returned to graduate school a year ago. Both my husband and I are in therapy; hopefully this counseling, plus attending a clinic for sexual disfunctions will enable us to remain married. But if not, I think we will both be at the point that we can survive divorce, and come through the whole experience with some positive gains.

Fantasy 1: My therapist (who is female) has arranged for me to be sexually counseled by a male friend, also a therapist. I meet regularly with him, once a week, in his apartment. He is very perceptive and sensitive; in the beginning, we only talk. He is very slow to introduce sexual activities. The second time I am there, he merely has me lie fully clothed next to him. It's as though he always sensed at what point the fears I have regarding sex negate the excitement, and always takes me on one step beyond where I think it's okay, but one step short of what would scare me away. This is my sweetest, gentlest fantasy, and I haven't yet gotten us to the point of actually making love, and orgasm (which I am only able to achieve while masturbating in real life).

Fantasy 2: (This is wild.) The beginning part of this borrows and adapts part of a science-fiction novel I once read. There is some group of people who have instituted a colony of "superpeople" . . . beautiful, strong, intelligent, etc. (Naturally, they want me. Such egotism.) Anyway, they get their population by kidnapping desirable persons.

I'm kidnapped, and awaken in a sparsely furnished bedroom. For the next two weeks, someone comes each day and takes me for different types of tests—a thorough physical which I really enjoy, especially the rectal examination for cancer (I never had this, but someone once described it to me), I.Q. tests, physical stamina tests, tests for pain threshold, sexual desire thresholds (ie., they studied my physiological responses to sexual stimulus à la Masters and Johnson). What is turning me on, aside from the discreet experiences of pain, sexual stimuli, etc., is the feeling of someone or something knowing all of me in such intimate detail.

In the meantime, they are also carrying on at this place social-psychology-type experiments. After a few days of testing, I return to the room and see drapes parted so that I can see a man in a similarly furnished adjacent room—apparently he can't see me. Later (on a different day), we see one another and try to talk through the glass; all we are able to communicate is that neither of us understand where we are or what's going on.

Finally, usually the day I endure the pain threshold experiments, I return quite shaken to the room, and see that now there is a doorway in the wall, and I cross over to his room, where he comforts me and holds me. Sometimes we screw, sometimes not, but it is always a gentle act.

Sometime later, he returns from a similar experience, and I comfort him. The sexual turn-on for me lies in the various tests performed, but this man is still an essential part of the fantasy; it occurs to me that maybe he is the safe place I can return to when sexual feelings have become too strong and, therefore, frightening to me (it is the loss of control I fear).

I have a couple of other remarks:

1: I think for me it's true that certain fantasies stem from childhood. I can remember having feelings reading the parts of *Tom Sawyer* where the schoolmaster switched children. I was raised a very strict Catholic and would never allow my "sexual" thoughts in my head. But thoughts of spankings and pain, which turned me on, didn't fall into that category. because I was too young to recognize those pleasurable feelings as sexual, or at least sensual. Likewise, a movie scene in which a group of rough men were ordering a woman in a bar to undress or they'd kill her male friend (knife at his throat) turned me on at almost age twelve, and my rape-type fantasies have this theme. The force is never raw strength, but psychological domination, threat of what they might do to someone else who is there (a male friend of mine) if I don't go along.

2: I would like to believe that the domination desire stems from the freedom from guilt which that situation provides. I very much identified with the woman in your book who said that the domination thing grew as her involvement in women's lib grew . . . the same thing happened to me, and it seemed like such a contradiction: the more liberated I felt in my day-to-day life, the more I fell back on and needed my domination fantasies during sex. Perhaps women's lib helped me to believe in my right to sexual feelings and experiences, but it's too difficult to forget all that guilt at once . . . so domination lets me have the pleasure without the guilt.

3: I liked the distinction you suggested between pain for pain's sake and pain as an instrument of domination. As you noted of other people, real pain turns me off; in fact, torture scenes in movies, etc., have made me upset to the point of nausea. I can't stand to hear people screaming, etc. But the thought of my bare ass being spanked as a preliminary to sex really turns me on, especially as the means by which a male forces me to suck him (which I have ambivalent feelings about, but am really turned off at the thought of doing it till he comes . . . something I've never done).

4: I found that fantasies of faceless people and unknown environments never made me feel guilty. But thinking of someone else I *know* while screwing with my husband still does, possibly because our marriage is not all that secure right now. However, I don't feel as cheap and shitty as I used to, having read in your book how many women do think of other men.

Thanks. I don't have the nerve to sign this with my real name. If any of the comments are helpful to you, let them be my way of contributing something in return for what I gained reading *My Secret Garden.*

Bonnie

Thank you for the first book. I couldn't believe how turned on I could get by reading, and ever since, I use your book to arouse myself before masturbating. Sure, I've got fantasies, *lots* of them! I'm twenty-one, lost my virginity at nineteen to someone who fell in love with me, have had sex with maybe seven or eight guys, no serious relationships, and over one hundred forty "dates" and casual affairs. I discuss sex and fantasies with my Mom and turned her on to your book (as well as EVERY woman I know). I love sex, anytime, anywhere, and am in the beginning of a beautiful relationship with an incredible guy who is a fabulous lover and who is very open about everything.

The one fantasy which started when I was about ten, has become a well-developed, detailed, and (excrutiatingly) arousing little plot that I embellish whenever I want to. However, the theme is always domination, and I always get spanked. One important detail is that the guy is smoking cigarettes—I guess this adds to his *macho* appearance. I only go out with very sensitive men who are in the creative field, but they've all been fairly dominating (but in a gentle, considerate way). I won't take shit from any guy and refuse to be told what to do. However, enough autobiography, here it is:

I am reading a book in his bed, wearing a fly-front skirt, button-down shirt, and only underpants. He comes in wearing jeans, a denim shirt, open very low down, and with a fitted leather jacket (collar up, of course). He comes over to the bed, sits down next to me, and tells me to put the book away. I refuse. He puts out his cigarette and takes the book out of my hand. *Everything* is done slowly, especially the stamping out of his many cigarettes, which elongates the fantasy and arouses me even more. I play innocent and do nothing except yawn or consistently refuse. He lights up another cigarette and makes a telephone call to his agent (he's an illustrator), and while on the phone unbuttons my shirt and takes it off. He rolls me over on my stomach and very slowly lifts up my skirt and pulls down my underpants and leaves me like that while he leaves the room to get a number for his agent. (As he puts the phone down, he whispers, "If you move, I feel sorry for you, and you can forget about sitting down for tonight.") When he comes back, I have sat up, pulled up my underwear, and pulled down my skirt. He hangs up and makes me stand in front of him while he sits at the edge of the bed and takes off my skirt. As I stand in front of him in just my underpants, he makes another phone call. While on the phone, he grabs me and puts me over his knee (by this time I probably have come about twenty times) and slowly pulls down my underpants. After the call, he spanks me very hard, but I refuse to cry. Then he fingers me while he makes another call, which lasts for maybe twenty minutes. After that one, he spanks me again, always in between each slap saying what a spoiled brat I am and how I've had this coming to me for a long time. He continues until I cry. Then he tells me to lay down and wait for him. He goes into the kitchen and comes back with rope and ties me up. He takes off his leather jacket, and rolls up his sleeves (this turns me on even more) and *teases* me for a long time (I love to be teased), then he unties me, and we make love all night, but he NEVER apologizes.

My thighs are locked together as I write this, and I'm trying to figure out how to get my boyfriend to do it. He has spanked me, but not long enough and not slowly; he also said he would act out my fantasies.

Hope this has helped, although I don't see how it could, it's too typical! Thanks again.

P.S. I'm an art student.

Sophie

Just wanted to let you know how much I enjoyed your book, *My Secret Garden*. I am twenty-five, single, and have had numerous lovers, all male. I have a master's degree in French and am a teacher by profession.

I have been fantasizing sexually since I was about five or six, when I began to masturbate. I was always ashamed of my fantasies—they were my private secret—up until about two or three years ago, when I underwent therapy with a psychiatrist. He practically had to drag these fantasies out of me—I didn't feel comfortable enough to tell him about them until I had been in therapy for close to two years. When I finally did tell him, I felt great relief that he accepted them and didn't recoil in horror and disgust when he heard them. Since that time, I have become much more relaxed about masturbating itself, enjoying it much more than before (now I can honestly *admit* that it is pleasurable), and I now also realize that sexual fantasies aren't dirty and disgusting, that indeed practically all women have them. I still masturbate regularly and enjoy that sort of "naughty" or even "dirty" feeling that used to repulse me. I also like to feel naughty and dirty when I'm screwing.

I realize that if I had not undergone therapy, I might never have discovered how pleasant and natural such fantasies can be, and that guilt feelings are not a necessary psychological "payment" for such pleasurable, but forbidden, thoughts. I hope that by reading your book, other women will draw the same conclusions about their fantasies, without the aid of a psychiatrist.

Thank you for your outstanding contribution to the liberation of the female sexual psyche.

I think I may attach some of my own fantasies to this letter. You may use them as you wish.

P.S. I read your book while at work (I'm doing temporary secretarial work during the summer) and beat off *three* times yesterday during the day, right at my desk!! Once I almost got caught, and it was ever so exciting!!

Fantasy 1: This one's an oldtimer—I used to use it exclusively, but now I usually use variations on the same theme, two of which also follow.

I am walking in the woods, enjoying the green scenery (I'll bet the shrink would say this is like walking through pubic hair), when all of a sudden I fall through a hole in the ground into a sort of laboratory. Inside the laboratory are lots of men in white coats (I guess they're doctors or something). I am undressed, weighed, and then put on some sort of cart which wheels me around to the various departments in the laboratory. First, I am examined and proclaimed healthy (internally, that is), and then the doctors determine that I am orgasmic and suitable for experimentation. The last stop is a big room with a kind of observation balcony. There are lots of men up there watching me, all extremely interested in so lovely a specimen as myself. The head doctor, or whatever he is, comes on the loudspeaker and announces that the gentlemen will soon witness a female orgasm. Then a large man comes in—he's usually very strong-looking, and although he's not physically dirty, he is perspiring and has a gleam in his eye that tells me he's going to do a job on me. This man has been trained by the lab, so that he knows precisely how to drive a woman into crazed ecstasy. I am strapped onto a table, my legs wide apart. The big man approaches me, explores me with his finger, smiles wickedly, nods in approval to the head doctor and the men observing the scene, then comes down on me, flicking my clit with his tongue. The whole time this is going on, the doctor is giving a blow-by-blow account of how I'm feeling and how turned on I'm getting over the loudspeaker. He tells the men that I'm getting very close to coming. Finally, the big man sucking my cunt can't stand it anymore himself, and so he drops his trousers, revealing a large, erect dick, and he fucks me for all he's worth, while at the same time flicking my clit with his finger, until I come, come, come, all over the fucking table.

Fantasy 2: This one has the same setting (sometimes I skip the beginning part and just find myself in the large room I described above). Now the men who were observing before are taking turns trying to turn me on, all this happening under the head doctor's watchful and approving eye. Each man tries his own special technique for exciting me, and the all-knowing doctor can tell who does the best job on me. The men try hard, because they know what the prize of doing the best job is—me (who else?). At some point, the doctor tells one of the men he has won me. This man then wheels the table I'm strapped to into another room, where he uses his technique to bring me to explosive orgasm by sucking, feeling, and fucking me.

Fantasy 3: Again the same background, except that now I've been at this laboratory for some time and know what to expect. I have come to enjoy this experimentation so much that, this time, the doctor announces over the loudspeaker, I have begged him to let someone work me over again. Same scene, same ending, except that this time I asked for it.

I just want to add that these are all fantasies that I use while masturbating. I don't normally fantasize too much while fucking, except that if someone's eating me out, I'll usually use one of these old standbys. I love to be fucked from behind while having my clit manipulated, either by me or my partner, and lots of times I can't come unless someone's playing with my clit. At any rate, I have my best orgasms when someone's fucking me and playing with my clit at the same time.

Dr. John Harrison

As you can see by the letterhead above (which I must ask you not to reprint, for obvious reasons), I am a psychoanalyst. This letter is to tell you that your book, *My Secret Garden*, is already having highly beneficial spinoffs in my therapeutic practice. For example, a young mother says, "I can't reveal my sexual fantasies to you directly but if you will look on page xx in Nancy Friday's book, you will read one that is something like mine!" As you might guess, by the conclusion of therapy, I hope she will be able to talk to me directly about all her sexual fantasies in complete detail. That would denote self-acceptance, maturity, responsibility, *and a giant step toward a more fulfilling life.*

Your book provides a most welcome generalizing example that encourages people to come to terms with themselves and perhaps seek some of the excitement of which they dream. *It is known, for example, that people with true psychosomatic illnesses, such as ulcers, hypertension, etc., are sadly lacking in the capacity to fantasize.* If they can learn to fantasize, their nervous stress, strain, anxiety, and frustration may be given an outlet in that manner, and not have to be expressed as destructive forces within their own poor bodies.

One other comment: many neurotics are entirely unconscious of their most important sexual fantasies. Psychoanalysis helps them make these conscious and acceptable. Most people are genuinely unaware of what really excites them, but from your "catalog" (if I may use such a shorthand term), they can find one very similar to their own previously unrecognized fantasies. In psychoanalysis, we find again and again that this basic fantasy had once been known and treasured, but then repressed out of shame, etc. I would compare your book to a jukebox with old, forgotten favorite tunes which, when played, bring back all the feelings of yesteryear.

Please continue with your good work. I know it must be pleasurable; I hope it is profitable. Now that you know that in the experience of at least one psychoanalyst, it is therapeutic as well, you must feel you have found the best of all occupations.

Your photo on the dust jacket does invite me to tell you a sexual fantasy of my own. You have an intimate, sexual, and candid look about you. Perhaps your appearance invites people to be candid with you in return. To tell such a fantasy is a mild sexual experience in itself—but you asked for it.

It is this: On any given day in my office, when a woman comes in with a brief miniskirt and no panties, she is rewarded with a gentle, moist, caressing of her cunt with my tongue. It would be important for her to sense that this would happen only if she gave a sign of acquiescence by the way she dressed and sat.

Freud talked about the sexual fantasies that patients had about their doctors, and went on to posit and discuss the countertransference this developed in their therapists. Which is a stuffy, polysyllabic word for what amounts to a little cunt-licking in my case.

I am sure you understand why I request that while you let the fact that I am a psychoanalyst stand, I ask that you assign me a fictitious name.

Deedee

I'm writing this because I think I may be a lesbian—I'm not sure. I think it all started when I was six or seven years old. My playmate and I used to take off all our clothes. Then I would climb on top of her (I'm very aggressive), open her pussy lips, and grind the hell out of her. Then I met her older sister, Tish. One day, Tish was alone in the house, and asked me to come over. She had on a nightgown, but with nothing underneath. She raised the gown and told me to rub her pussy. I did it, and in my fantasies even today, I am often still seven years old. I like to remember how I opened her lips and tickled her clitoris. Even as I write this, I can imagine how she looked when she reached climax. The reason I think I may be a lesbian is that she didn't tell me to open her pussy lips and tickle her. I did this all on my own.

When I became eight years old, I gave up my playmate for a boyfriend named Teddy. Teddy and I used to go down into the basement and take off all our clothes and fuck all day. (I know that isn't the way it could have been. but that's how it seems in my memories.) But he soon told his pals, and they joined us. One day, seven boys pulled a train on me. I didn't tell my mom or dad, because I enjoyed it so much. But I think that incident is what made me dislike boys and want to go back to women.

When I say "Go back to women," I mean, thinking about them, fantasizing about them. I often find myself wanting to have an affair with a woman rather than a man. As I've said earlier, I am very aggressive. When I go out with a nice man, I find myself being bossy. I like to make up fantasies about girls with blonde hair and blue eyes. (I am black.) In my fantasies, I always see myself going up to them on the street and propositioning them. But in real life, I never do. I also want to rape my best friend. I think I'm waiting for the right moment. She doesn't know the real me. I've never told her how I feel about her, and the part she plays in my fantasies. Perhaps I will grow out of this phase. Maybe I don't know very much about life since I'm only seventeen. and want to shock my parents. Am I really mixed up, or is this a super, superfantasy?

P.S. To show you what thinking can do, even though I have not described my fantasies in any complete way, I have been thinking about them while writing this, and my cunt is dripping wet!

Loretta

The idea of "innocence" being initiated into sexual pleasure and orgasm is something I love to use in fantasies, my favorite having to do with a "religious" experience. (Oddly enough, I had no religious upbringing, and no religious experiences of any kind.)

In the fantasy, I am a young girl who has been raised without any sexual knowledge. My family are church-

goers; I am meant to be pure and virginal. When I
reach the right age (late puberty), my parents take
me to church for some special religious instruction from
the "priest." He takes me alone into the room for
initiates. There are candles burning around a cushioned
table that is covered with purple velvet. The priest wears
long robes. He is a man in his thirties or forties, with
a quality of masculine virility, despite presumed celibacy.
He has a deep voice. He explains that I am now to un-
dergo a very holy condition—the supreme ecstasy of God's
greatest power. I will experience extraordinary sensations,
quite beyond anything I've ever known, but I must freely
open my will, and my body, to the holy spirit. I must
allow myself to react without fear to whatever frenzied
state the holy spirit ordains when it takes possession of
me. And I must be in the pure state of complete nudity.
"Don't be embarrassed now; this is a holy thing that
is about to happen to you. . . ." He helps me remove
my clothing and instructs me to lie down on the cushioned
table so that he may prepare both my soul and body.
While I lie naked on the table, he anoints my breasts,
belly, thighs, with perfumed oil, and intones prayers and
chants. "Let this young woman be filled with the holy
spirit. Enter her body and soul and encompass her in
the greatest ecstasy. Fulfill her in joyous holiness. . . ."
His touch is pleasant, strangely provocative, and
mysterious. His voice is hypnotic. I lie in an entranced
stupor. He waves a scepter over me. It is made of gold,
with a rounded, bulblike tip. "Let the holy scepter find
the entrance to her soul through her body . . ." he
murmurs. He lays the round gold top on my throat, my
shoulders. . . . Every place he touches produces a magic
tingling—probing my breasts, nipples, stroking my belly.
It moves toward my loins. Cool metal stroking between
my labia. The sensation produces a soft moan from me,
an uncontrolled lift of my torso. "Ah," says the priest.
"This must be where we will find the magic orifice . . .
the pathway of the holy spirit." He opens my body with
the metal scepter. It slides into me, filling an orifice of

my body that I never knew I had until now. . . . "Yes, it is here!" he cries. "Do you feel it . . . the beginnings of your experience of ecstasy? Is the holy spirit beginning to work in you?"

"Yes . . . yes. I think so. . . ."

"You must give in to it, my dear. You must give in completely to whatever feelings the holy spirit creates as it takes possession of you. . . . You will give in?"

I nod, and groan. The scepter slides in and out; as it slides in, it fills me with unexplainable excitement. My body moves in reaction, out of my control.

"Do you think it is coming? Do you feel the holy spirit coming to you?"

"Yes . . . yes!"

"Let it come . . . however it wishes. . . ."

The priest is doing something unexpected, but I am too overcome to be concerned at the moment. The table has a drop leaf at the end, which he lowers so that he can move himself up closer to me, between my legs. With a quick movement, he opens the lower front of his robes, and brings out another scepter. As the metal scepter pulls out of me, he pushes the other one in, leaning over me, his face contorted with ecstasy, too. it would seem. Perhaps we are both meant to be fulfilled with the holy spirit together. He presses his other magic scepter deep inside me. It feels smooth and warm, and extraordinarily tantalizing. "Is it coming?" he cries.

"Yes . . . something is happening to me!"

"Let it come! Do what it wants you to do!"

It is making my body writhe and undulate. My orifice swallows and squeezes his scepter with a sensation that is driving me into a wild, delicious frenzy. Never have I felt anything like this. . . . The holy spirit is about to overcome me. I can feel it! He acknowledges my groans and thrashings with, "Yes . . . yes! That is it! Here it comes! It is here!"

(Amen and hallelujah! You bet your sweet scepter, your holiness . . . you have made it come, and it has come to you, too, you devil you. . . .)

I return to the priest and the room of initiation time and time again. I receive more instruction and more experience in the ways of being entered and fulfilled by the holy spirit. I am a devout young woman. . . . With the candles burning and the scepter sliding into me, I experience, time and time again, the greatest of all religious ecstasies. The priest and my parents rejoice in my religious gifts. Sometimes the priest shows me paintings of the saints having religious experiences—naked bodies in the midst of ecstasy—arched backs, contorted faces. I may wonder how these physical experiences can actually relate to the soul. Secretly, I begin to doubt the authenticity of the priest and the validity of this "church." I think he is a bit of a fraud. Even the most innocent have some concept of sexuality. But I never let on; never mention my suspicions. I am having far too much fun to give it up; and everyone (except perhaps the priest himself) believes me a thoroughly pure, devout, innocent, and religious young woman. . . . We pretend, and fool each other, and continue to have glorious orgasms on the purple table.

Sharon

Having read your book, I decided to write to you and tell you my fantasies.

First, let me tell you a little about myself. I am a thirty-five-year-old virgin (also Virgo!) and relatively happy under the circumstances.

My divorced mother and twice-divorced grandmother live with me—my mother is sixty-four (today!), and my grandmother, who cannot walk, is eighty-six. Both are in poor health, and I don't expect them to live long.

My mother hates sex, and her attitude caused her twenty-year marriage to come to an end when I was ten years old. I was "word blind," but overcame this and finally graduated from the University of Ohio.

Presently, I work in a library where through reading

have "liberated" my own attitude toward sex. Actually, I realized how sick my mother's attitude was long ago.

As a child, I enjoyed sex-play with several boys who lived close by me, and recoved from my guilt while studying Freud in high school.

I am a Methodist and a Republican, and I *do* believe more and more in the new morality.

I attend church for social reasons, but disregard the Pauline letters and believe in the occult sciences (I love to cast horoscopes!).

Starting with my present fantasies—I found in my student-teaching that I was VERY attracted to young boys. One of them, a bisexual, used to come to my house (before my grandmother's illness) while my mother worked We spent the day in bed "necking." I gave him photos of nude people from *Playboy* on which I glued male sex organs—aimed at the females. I got these pictures from *Sexology* magazine.

We would look at the photos—he was seventeen and I was twenty-eight—and become aroused. We would kiss and breathe. Then he would masterbate under the covers or go to the bathroom. Finally, he would leave—go to the bus station and "make it" with a boy. We played this game day after day. Our pleasure was to hold out. He wouldn't even bring a rubber so I would be afraid to "let him" in case he would get me pregnant. He and I both loved to know how much we wanted each other—but neither would give over to the passion.

Many times when I was breathing hard, he would lie on me and watch me struggle to not give in. Sometimes, I was on him watching his face while he tried to get his hands to his penis in order to jerk off.

Finally. we both got tired of our game and just drifted apart with NO hard feelings.

I believe we BOTH enjoyed being wanted by another and JUST leaving it that way.

My fantasies stem from this experience.

Fantasy 1: We do live together, as my "family" have all died. He discovers I need more sex, and I want it from boys in their early teens and inexperienced. He loves money so he gathers heterosexual boys once a week to come to "our" house (they pay him).

I am now completely nude with my legs wide and far apart—there are about six boys partly dressed (pants on) standing around the bed.

George (my lover and former student) helps a boy about twelve "mount" me.

I can feel his young penis move into me—then he starts to move faster and faster. The room is silent.

One at a time, these boys "learn to be men" using my body. But only until George enters me do I have a climax.

Fantasy 2: A short fantasy—I set up a movie camera, and we have home movies of ourselves having intercourse.

Fantasy 3: I bathe George in the tub and then rub him down with powder and oils. We then have intercourse.

Fantasy 4: George has a date with a young girl—she won't let him sleep with her—he comes home to my front door—it is dark and his penis (very large) is out of his pants—we make love on the sofa in the living room. He never leaves me again.

Fantasy 5: We decide to have a child, so I hire a real good prostitute to live with us to take care of his sex drive. After he has had intercourse with her, he comes to bed with me, and I examine him to see if he is relaxed and soft. Then we go to sleep.

Fantasy 6: Sometimes he has to have a boy for sexual release, so I give him money to go to the bus station to get what he wants.

Fantasy 7: Most of my fantasies are just having relations with him.

Fantasy 8: Sometimes I think it would be fun to go to the basement of the library and have oral sex with him—while everyone is having a coffee break in the next room.

Fantasy 9: Sometimes I dream (awake) of having oral sex (I don't care for it performed on myself) with him lying on his back. I watch his face as he feels great pleasure.

Whenever I am interested in someone or date them, I have fantasies about them—I do NOT masturbate with my fantasies—(much) maybe twice a year! I always wonder about the size of a man's penis—almost EVERY man I meet. Yet I have NEVER seen a man's penis except in photos (to me they are beautiful!).

My fantasies take place normally in the morning!

Sometimes at night (I usually go right to sleep!) and many times at the library.

My sex drive is stronger a day or so before my period. Just being around young men (in their twenties) will "turn me on."

I almost always respond to my fantasies and photos of nude men by getting very wet.

If I am around "George"—a few days before my period, have been looking at photos (nudes), the wetness goes down my legs, and I pull and tug.

People would be surprised to know that while I speak to them on the street—I am "opening up" and ready to have relations.

As a young teenager, I dreamed of having relations with black men and animals. Just recently have tired of the thought of having relations with monkeys.

I have tried fantasies with women, but it seems too silly to continue.

Ms. Friday, I don't believe in marriage—I think it is rotten for all concerned. I plan to live with men, whom I really want, at the death of both mother and grandmother.

I get along very well with men and am popular!! So don't let Helen Gurley Brown tell you that virgins are not attractive nor popular. Nuts.

I allow men to discuss sex with me. But I refuse to be insulted with dirty jokes.

Because I really like men AS PEOPLE and accept their sex drive—I am a popular virgin.

Many of the nonvirgins have made fun of me at work (I never say I am a virgin to anyone, but they seem to know it) only to have the new men and boys employed at the library go AFTER me. It serves them right! Ha.

Also, I accept my own sexual drive—enjoy it—BUT I refuse to let it destroy my life.

I am enclosing my photo so you can SEE a thirty-five-year-old virgin! And a FAIRLY happy one at that.

Good luck with your research—because of people like you—I know I am not alone with my "dreams."

☐ In Brenda's fantasy, which follows, she uses words in a very special way: to heighten her erotic moments. While the sexual act is going on, Brenda verbally describes it to herself, making a running commentary on events that one would think are so vivid they would leave nothing to be described at all. This internal monologue is, I feel, another layer of sexuality: while her lover is exciting her body, Brenda's verbal description to herself becomes a fantasy that excites her mind, making sex itself more real to her . . . one more example of the idea that the mind is the most powerful sexual organ of all. ☐

Brenda

I am twenty-one, a musician, and gay.

I loved your book, *My Secret Garden,* and congratulate you on your bravery.

The first sexual fantasy I can remember is vague, but it had something to do with bugs (the little black pill bugs that roll up when you poke them) crawling on my clit. (I was only about two or three). When I was sixteen, and was in love, I used to dream of sucking his cock all day at school! And I would suck it every chance I got in reality. After about a year, he was gone, and I began to fantasize about my best girl friend who was twenty-two and was a "bad girl." (She had a couple illegit babies, abortions, etc.) When I slept with her, I couldn't sleep at all, thinking of how beautiful she was, and how any guy would love to be in bed there next to her. (My real sex life was limited to hetero.)

We went our separate ways, and when I was nineteen, my new best girl friend would come to see me, and we'd talk about sex and get ourselves all worked up, and then we'd have a hard time sleeping. I would think of how I'd like to run the tips of my fingers lightly over her vagina walls and clit! And touch her clit lightly again and again with my finger.

Eventually, we acted out our fantasies, and she swears it was the best orgasms she ever had; however, she is now back with men (for social reasons, strict upbringing, etc.).

I have had five affairs with women (from fifteen to twenty-three) that have lasted longer than my hetero-sexual affairs lasted. (I have had about thirty men before discovering my preference.)

I found my hetero experiences sexually unsatisfying. While my girl friends get me off every time. Though once when this girl I dug was going down on me, I had to envision the one girl I wanted more eating me before I could come.

I like young girls (not really young, about sixteen), and when they go down on me, I think "That beautiful long hair, and lovely graceful body; she's sucking me. Now she's inserting her fingers in and out of me, and it feels better than the biggest cock." When I am the aggressor, I think of what will make her feel good; what I like, or if she'll tell me and show me what she likes, I concentrate on this.

Gena

I wish first to compliment you on *My Secret Garden*. It is truly what I believe to be the *first* book to take the giant step toward really understanding female sexuality. It deals candidly, openly, and honestly with women.

I should acquaint you with myself before I make my own contribution to your next book. I am nineteen, married two-and-a-half years, and soon to be a mother for the second time. I consider myself oversexed—if there is such a thing!—and bisexual. I hope I have gained a wider-than-average acquaintance over the past few years with life, love, sex, and the self-improvement arts.

I can remember that my fantasies began at an early age; five or six. At this age, I would often think how very nice it would feel to have someone older do these "naughty, but oh so nice," things to me . . . as I lay in my bed, night after night, riding a tightly stretched piece of sheet with my tiny "cunny." In particular, I hoped it would happen with a seventeen-year-old boy who was a neighbor. I also couldn't wait to know what a boy's "thingy" looked and felt like. Then one day, in the spring following my seventh birthday, all my fantasies were answered. Terry (I remember him well) asked me to join him in "listening to some music." The stereo was in his room, which was actually a bunkhouse well away from his parent's house and the rest of their farm. When we began talking, I soon felt we had become close, and so I thought it would be "proper" for me to ask him some pretty personal questions. He seemed to get a strange gleam in his eyes and said, "Shoot!" I remember the first and only question I had a chance to ask that day was, "What do boys look like down there?" He made me promise not to tell a soul, and then asked if I really would like to see for myself—that would be easier than trying to explain, he said. I very anxiously said yes. He

66

took down his clothes and stood before me. I remember staring at his penis and wanting so badly to touch it. He sensed it. "You want to touch me, don't you?" he said. "Take off your jeans, and I'll show you how nice we can feel." Again, I anxiously did so. He then "felt me up" until I almost died because it only kept feeling better and better. Then he showed me how to "bring him off." How delightful that first experience was, and I doubt it will ever be forgotten.

Through age ten, I continued having more and more sexual adventures, but about that age, I began to have fantasies about what it would be like to hold and be held by another of my own sex. At age eleven, I found out.

My parents were good friends with another local dairy family, and the children of both families got on well. In fact, they were the favorite playmates of my brother, sister, and myself, and we would often spend entire weekends together. They were our ages exactly. Marie and myself were the eldest at eleven, R. (my brother) and Ted were nine, and C. (my sister) and Rosalie were eight.

Both Marie and I felt funny in the world of children by then, as we were both wearing size 34B bras, and each had a healthy bush. We had often told one another about out sexual encounters and curiosities on the subject. So one evening when we were in bed in her room (during one of our stays), I initiated our mutual "female body" curiosities. But I did it only after I thought she was asleep. I reached around to her breasts (she was lying with her backside to my tummy) and began touching them ever so gently so as not to awaken her. But soon she was breathing heavily and moaning softly. I froze, knowing these as a sign of sexual excitement. Softly, I called out her name. She answered with "What?" in the same soft voice. All I could say were what turned out to be the two most beautiful words I would say for years to come: "Touch me!"

She did it, and we then proceeded and spent the rest of the night caressing one another's bodies with both hands and mouths, although we did not know about cunnilingus: that was the only act we did not perform on one another.

I grew to puberty with fantasies of lesbian affairs, but also what it would feel like to have a man. Then in 1969, I met the men who is now my husband. We lost our virginity to one another.

When I got married, my fantasies stopped until September or October of 1972, after six months of marriage and the birth of our daughter. Our marriage began to fall apart, and we separated a year later. He left me with our daughter and went back to Washington State where he was born, and where we had made our first home. I remained in Arizona, which had been our second home.

The fantasy that I began having in October of 1972 would be to think of meeting one of two types of fellows. One was Indian, easy-going, very considerate. He would be willing to learn and experiment in sex. Above all, he would have great control, so our sex could go on for hours. We would have no problems, no jealousy or embarrassments.

The other fellow would also be an Indian, but very rich, huge in structure, and very carefree in a kind of crazy way. I would be satisfied with him sexually because of his willingness to give wholly of himself, and his size; also because he would introduce me to sexual trios.

As fantastic as it may sound, in the two months that my husband and I were seperated, I *did* meet these two types. I formed a very loving relationship with them both; yet it was definitely not the kind of love I had for my husband.

When my husband and I reunited after our separation, I felt better, because I had lived out my fantasies, fulfilling them. I had my shit together, and we both felt our relationship would be better than it had ever been. We have become much more open and honest with one another and are now expecting the result—our second child.

I now see my husband in a new light sexually,

physically, and mentally. I bring myself to a mind-blowing climax in masturbating or sex with him by thinking about his beautiful body and how good he is to me. I can honestly say that with him life couldn't be better!

Although I am satisfied with him as I've just said, honesty does make me admit that I often fantasize still about other women (and truly wish it would happen on a more adult basis). I have a friend who might share these wishes for a sexual encounter, and I often wish she would, but I never talked to her about it at any length. I think of giving her as much pleasure as I possibly could with both my hands and mouth. The idea of going down on her excites me tremendously! Then after I have fulfilled her completely, she would in turn give me the same beautiful pleasures. It would be so good for both her and me, because who could possibly please a woman better than another? Who knows better what it feels like? I would definitely do it if the opportunity arose.

Much good luck to you on your second book.

Joyce

I've just completed reading your book, *My Secret Garden.* When I saw your address in the back of the book and the request for comments, I felt compelled to write. I'm now a college grad, age twenty-two, and was first turned on to the wonder of having sex only one year ago. My first and still current lover is a sexual dynamo. He can keep it up and going strong for as long as one hour, in which I have so many orgasms that I lose count. I don't fantasize while we're fucking, because I have such a tremendous time enjoying the good fuck. Basically, I read your book for more ideas to vary my sex life, and to bring more enjoyment to my lover and myself. Whatever I think of, I make a point of putting into reality, but tonight, my lover is out of town on business, so I must resort to fantasizing in memory that we are doing some of the things together we have done in the past.

These are the fantasies I had tonight. My middle name to my boyfriend is Linda Lovelace. Needless to say, I am now considered a pro at this technique, and I imagined that I am eating his whole cock by getting it down my whole throat as far as I can to overcome the gagging reflex. I have a beautiful mouthful of saliva which I use to further wet his lovely cock, balls, and inner thighs. I also thought of a scene in which he was fucking me from behind. While in this doggy position I bend my head so as to watch him fuck me. He is doing various things too, like, "Look, ma—no hands." He is also fondling my breasts as I massage his massive balls, and I can see and touch his beautiful cock as it moves in and out of my cunt.

My boyfriend is also the greatest lover for me (I have had three other men, by the way). For example, he will lick and kiss my cunt and suck my clitoris. Then he sticks his tongue up my wet, juicy cunt (that's what he calls it, "juicy") and makes like he's fucking me with his tongue. I just love this.

Writing all this down has resulted in my cunt becoming soaking wet and ready for action. But alas, I must hold tight until I'm with my lover again, and we can make up for lost time.

So to all of you out there—Get Fucked (and have a Ball doing it!).

P.S. I think that what makes all my sexual activity so enjoyable to me is that my parents were so strict with me when I was growing up. I was the last virgin in my crowd of friends, and was always very fearful of what people would say if they "found out." So you can imagine what great pleasure I felt when I came to sex, late as I did, and found it was so marvelous, instead of being the frightening thing my parents wanted me to feel.

CHAPTER TWO

ADOLESCENCE

☐ With the advent of menstruation, childhood ends, adolescence begins. We are suddenly thrown into a larger world than we feel prepared for, given more choices than childhood ever offered. Much as we longed to be thought mature and adult, now that it has begun at last, we suffer role and identity confusions. "What are you going to be when you grow up?"—the question throws us into despair. We wanted to do one thing yesterday, but that's no longer true today, and we suspect we will change our minds again tomorrow. Above all, we want to say, "I don't know. I'm too young to make up my mind." But that's not allowed. Only *kids* can say that. Instead, we lapse into sulky silence or give top-of-the-head answers. The pressures of family and society, the mandates of an educational system that rushes us on express rails into the future seem to give us no pause to rest and think about who we are.

It is at this age that we begin to fall in love—over and over again. While this is obviously an expression of our growing sexual maturation, it is also an expression of our search for identity: one of the great wonders of first love is how each new man seems to help us find a new person within ourselves.

For this reason, I think it is unfortunate that contemporary mores demand that love be certified by sex. It may not really be what the young girl wants yet. Sex itself can become one more force pushing her ahead too far, too fast, in a direction she is not yet sure she wants to take. "I love you," she wants to say to him, but is afraid: it may be the final signal he needs to open the door to the bedroom. *Put up or shut up.* She may or may not want sex right now, but what she does want, desperately, is for him to speak. She wants him to say he loves her too so that she can ask him to describe this woman he loves. Who is she? What is so wonderful about her? Is she really *me?* She has a sense of unreality about herself; she needs to find herself reflected in someone else's affectionate eye, shaped and formed there into an image of herself she can see and understand. She has been looking into mirrors too long. "Tell me the kind of girls you like," we ask the young men we know. *Tell me how to be.* A little shiver runs through me every time I hear that request in a young woman's voice, no matter what the actual words are. It is *the* ontological question, a search for a base upon which to build our being. We look to each other for clues, but it is a question we all must answer in our own time, in our own way. What makes "plastic people" not ring true is that they have not listened within for an answer; they have built their conforming, counterfeit selves out of the meretricious junk that society has handed them. Dr. R. D. Laing (*The Divided Self*) finds this question at the very heart of schizophrenia—or perhaps, the lack of an answer to it. The job of creating our authentic identity is one of the great tasks of adolescence.

It is why teenagers spend so much of their emotional energy and time in talk: it is all work toward definition. In their endless speculations about eternity, truth, beauty, good, and evil—just as in their giggly bits of gossip—they are uncovering layers of personality, assaying for the gold of their true selves. One of the most hopeful developments of our time, I feel, is that young women no longer listen only to young men for clues of who they are. We ask that question today of other women too, each one of us strengthening every other in our determination to define our sex for ourselves—and not merely in terms of what it is supposed men want. The Great Male Buyer's Market is over; we will no longer sell ourselves out.

Fantasies that arise out of the crises of adolescence are characterized by trying on different personalities, testing various likes and dislikes, rehearsing our sexuality for events that are yet to come. Sis proudly tells us in her letter that she is an A-student in school. But immediately she feels she must fight the goody-goody definition this seems to bestow upon her by telling us she has "a very strong sex drive and wants to make love." Does she? Or is this merely one of the okay things girls of her age feel they must say? (Just as their mothers, a generation earlier, felt they had to say the opposite.) When the opportunity for sex is actually presented to Sis by a boy she knows well and who promises to be "very gentle" with her, she literally jumps up in alarm and cries, "I won't!"

I am very sympathetic to young women like Sis. Despite all their brave talk, something deep within them knows they aren't ready for sex. Sis doesn't know why this is true. She is not reinforced by her peers—everyone around her seems to take sex for granted. She is alone with only her feelings to guide her—*but they are enough*. She doesn't have to know why she is not yet ready for sex; she only has to be in touch with her feelings: her body informs her mind, and her answer is *no*. I applaud her for going along with her gut reaction, particularly so because it is a self-determined response at odds with what seem to be the accepted slogans and ideas of her friends. Our lifelong struggle is to teach our reason and emotions to move in tandem on the same tides. Just as I believe every woman has the right to say *yes* if she feels like it—and is willing to take the responsibility for her actions—so has she the perfect right to refuse, if the mysterious ebb and flow of desire is not yet upon her.

In the fantasies that Sis sends us, we see that she is getting ready for the truly sexual time she knows lies ahead. But that time is not yet.

For Beth Anne, too, fantasies are exciting strategies for getting used to an idea about which she is still ambivalent. She tells us she is a virgin, and too shy to buy *My Secret Garden* at the bookshop where she works, even though she could get it there at a discount. In her fantasies, we see her other side: she is a woman who would like to have sex with "a customer, a stranger in the street, someone I don't know too well." And then she adds a sentence that reminds us how much she is like Sis. "Boy," writes Beth Anne, "when it does happen, I'll be really ready after all these rehearsals in my head."

Penelope's letter shows us another exploration of sexual identity through fantasy. The child of intelligent, permissive parents, she felt free enough with her mother to ask to be taught how to masturbate, after reading Masters and Johnson brought the idea to mind. In her letter, we see that she has grown into the kind of young woman we would expect from such a family: she is sexually knowing, sophisticated, one who feels free and secure enough to ask men out herself "occasionally," instead of always waiting passively to be asked. But in her fantasies, she explores a totally opposite identity, "the woman I can't let myself be (dumb, naïve, unaware of my sexuality). . . ."

Even if we had parents like Penelope's, something in us still wants to establish ourselves as people in our own right by rebelling against them. But when the parents are decent, reasonable, and intelligent people, rebellion itself becomes unreasonable; their very permissiveness is frustrating, giving us no firm base to push off against. But our negative emotions want to be expressed anyway. In fantasies like Penelope's, the problem is solved. She *is* the woman she "can't let myself be." That is, she is the *dumb broad* that her parents' training has made it impossible for her to be. She has circumvented them in her imagination: rebellion at last. □

Sis

I am young (fifteen) and a virgin. I have met many boys I like. but have never had sexual relations with any as far as making out. I think the reason for this is I am very shy. and I worry that boys are going to tell my friends what we do. I am an A-student in school and popular. and I don't want to spoil that, but I have a very strong drive and want to make love.

The latest turn down I made was while visiting some friends that live a long distance from my house (we have known them since they were small). One of their brothers' friends was my age and came over to see us. The brother's friend has a swimming pool. and they go there often. He invited us to go swimming that afternoon. So we did. When we were fixing to leave, they said they left a towel at the pool and for me to run and get it. The boy my age was there and no one else, while getting the towel. He said he liked me and to ask my friends that I was staying with to let me stay awhile to swim some more. They said yes. We swam awhile, and then we got out to get something to eat. His mother was on a trip, and he was staying by himself.

As we walked through the door, he put his arms around me from behind and began kissing my neck; I turned and kissed him and we made out on the sofa about fifteen minutes. but he was not satisfied. He escorted me upstairs to his bedroom and pulled off his swimming trunks while I was laying on the bed. I jumped and said, "I won't," and he said that he knew how I felt and would be very gentle with me. He said that all he wanted to do was show how much he liked me and only wanted to explore my body with his fingers and mouth and for me to do the same to him. that he didn't want to fuck unless I wanted to. I ran out of the room and called my friends to come and get me.

75

I often fantasize what would have happened if I hadn't run out. Here is the best one:

After long persuasion, I would not let him touch me. He says, "What if we go to the pool, get in up to our neck, then you take off your swimming suit, and I feel you, that way I won't be able to see you. . . ." I say okay.

We get in up to our neck, and he unfastens my top and slips it off, the same with the bottoms. He kisses me once and then slips his hand between my legs. He watches the expression on my face as he does. He clutches one of my breasts. He then separates the lips of my pussy and rubs his finger back and forth over my clitoris, stimulating me out of control. Then he takes his cock and slips it in between the lips rubbing it quickly as with his finger. I can't stand it any longer and beg him to suck me; still in the water, he lifts me up onto a raft with my legs hanging over in the water and my pussy at the edge, he sucks me vigorously and then slides his tongue as far as possible in my vagina. I then change places with him, this time he is on the raft. I take his cock in my mouth and suck hard. THE END.

When I was little, my cousin, a male, lived beside me. One day, he said he would check me himself so I wouldn't have to go to the doctor. I agreed because I hated to go to the doctor. He took off my clothes and did everything possible he could. He opened the lips of my pussy and felt, sucked, and licked them, then he made me do the same to him. He put an ice cube between my pussy, which drove me crazy. Then I told him I had to use the bathroom, so he stood me up, placed his mouth over my pussy, and I used the bathroom in his mouth. This delighted me more than ever. We did this many times up until I was eight. The first time he did it, I was four and he was seven.

Now the way I meet my sexual urges is to vibrate myself. I lay on the bed, pants off, vibrator between my legs for two to three minutes, and I stimulate myself to orgasm. It's a wonderful feeling; I think when I get up the courage to let a man do it, I will love it.

Beth Anne

Hello. I was already in bed (alone) and almost asleep when I got this urge to write to you!

I have just finished *My Secret Garden,* and I would like you to know that the book was one of the most informative and interesting ones I've ever read, and believe me, I read a lot.

I work in a bookstore here in Philadelphia. Your book arrived last week. Our manager, who was very staunchly and religiously brought up, was on vacation, so we all took turns leafing through the book. Our assistant manager (who incidentally is homosexual) told me the book was filthy. I'm seventeen; he's thirty-three. I picked the book up occasionally, halfway on the sly for a few days, and then last week, I bought it from a "rival" store, because I was too embarrassed to ask if it could be "stripped," or to write up the sale in the employee discount tablet.

What follows now is a conversation that took place between myself and the other salesperson, Tina, who is twenty-three, married, no kiddies. It took place when we were sort of slow and didn't have anything better to do than stand around and B.S.

Tina: Have we sold any *M.S.G.* yet?

Me: Yeah. a few, considering we just put them out.

Tina: Hmmm. . . .

Me: I bought a copy today downtown, 'cause I was a little nervous about buying it here.

Tina: Really? I'd love to read it when you're through. I said it was filthy because Jim [Asst. Mgr.] was there, and I figured he might get upset if I showed an interest. . . . I was also afraid Mary [Mgr.] might walk in, and I'd REALLY be embarrassed.

So you see, it's something that just about every woman is interested in, although it's probably considered more socially acceptable not to be.

The sexual fantasies I have now occur usually at night when it's quiet, and I have time to elaborate without being interrupted. I'm still a virgin, although I'm not so sure I want to be one that much longer. Just reading your book and thinking about the guy I'm in love with have made me think twice about resisting his advances. He's twenty-five, and really supernice, although I'm not sure if he'll be around much longer, and I'd kind of like my first sexual encounter to be with someone I truly love.

The funny thing is, when I'm dating someone I really care for, I never fantasize about them. It seems rather unfair to fantasize about them when I don't even know if they could live up to my fantasies in real life. I think I'd like to be surprised.

Usually, my thoughts center around a man I find fantastically attractive and very nice, i.e., a customer, a stranger on the street, someone I don't know too well. I can imagine him doing all sorts of things to me, all the things I've ever read about. And I can respond to him wholeheartedly, because there's no problem about what will happen afterward (he'll probably go away and just leave me totally satisfied). But, of course, what I really want is that these fantasies happen with a man I love. Boy, when it does happen, I'll be really ready after all these rehearsals in my head! When I meet that man, I can be drunk, stoned, angry, or happy, and so can he but as long as we love each other it will be all right. I suppose this is all because I am a basically insecure person and need to be assured of my attractiveness frequently.

All luck in your next book. We need it! Take care. Peace.

Penelope

At the end of your book, *My Secret Garden,* you ask for suggestions, comments, or more fantasies. I'd like to share some of my garden with you.

My earliest memory is when I was probably ten, or eleven. A friend and I had somehow discovered that her family's electric toothbrush when placed on a certain area, caused mysterious sensations. I didn't know what I was feeling, but I remember always taking the device off me when the extreme tenseness began. I never continued to what I know now as an orgasm.

Aside from the few weeks my friend and I escaped into the bathroom, I remember nothing sexual until I was fifteen. I was attempting to read Masters and Johnson's *Human Sexual Response* and asked my mother how to masturbate. She told me, and ever since then, I've enjoyed myself almost every night. That was seven years ago.

My early fantasies often started with me dancing around the bedroom, performing for a hidden audience of aroused men. Once in a while, a few were allowed to participate, and I'd rub my breasts against the cold mirror and manipulate my clitoris and eventually get back to the bed to come and collapse. Sometimes, especially when I first began masturbating, I'd time the "session" and see how quickly I could come.

Up until just a few months ago, I always stimulated my clitoris only. I never enjoyed simulating intercourse, because until recently, I never enjoyed it in reality. Even now my clitoris is the focus of my masturbating.

My present fantasies are very varied. (*My Secret Garden* helped me expand my nightly choices!) Sometimes the woman is aggressive, but mostly she is what I refer to as "the dumb broad." She is busty and naïve. She wears low-cut tops, but is unaware of the lustful glances she gets. Usually, she is conned into

79

drinking more than she should or smoking some powerful pot. She bends over and more boob comes out or a strap slips down, and the man continues to move in, slyly. Eventually, things get too hot for her to want to stop him. I never see my face in these fantasies. I either make up unknown people or use scenes from movies and the stars from those scenes. When the fantasy begins, the woman is not thinking SEX. The man is. And what first begins me getting high, my climb toward orgasm, is seeing the woman's chest; I am the man at this point in the fantasy. During the man's approach, I am both feeling the sensations of the woman's body and also getting excited as the man because of the progress toward and anticipation of getting this woman. When the actual fucking is about to begin, I am solely the woman, raising my hips, desperately anxious for that cock to enter and satisfy me.

You spoke often in your book of how fantasies are often expressions of what one would like to experience in reality. In analyzing my fantasies, I found it really interesting that the woman I can't let myself be (dumb, naïve, unaware of my sexuality) is exactly the woman who dominates my daydreams. In reality, I am never passive. I ask men out occasionally, make love when I want to (if the opportunity is present), and present myself as a whole person rather than a game-playing female. In some ways, I hate the fact that I get most excited when fantasizing the "dumb broad" role. I'm hoping someday to be close enough with a man to feel free and act out some of these fantasies. I'd like to see if they get me more excited, quicker than I actually get in reality. I'm usually too conscious and aware to let go and enjoy myself. Actually, in three years of fucking (not regularly all that time), I have come a few times from oral sex and once during intercourse, only when my clitoris was stimulated at the same time. I've rarely fantasized when with a man. (I plan to start though.) I always come when I masturbate.

I'd also just like to support your comments regarding

the sharing of fantasies. Because of my family's openness, I never felt strange or bad or guilty about my fantasies or masturbating. But I've talked to many friends who had never shared their experiences of masturbation or fantasies. And what a great experience to be talking to a friend about fantasies and find that we use the exact same scene from a book!

I thank you for your first book and hope your next is successful. Please feel free to use any of what I've written. I've enjoyed sharing it with you, and if there's anything else I might be able to write about to give you more material, please send me a note, and I'll get something to you. I enjoy thinking about sex and talking about myself.

Good luck.

☐ During the turmoil of our adolescent years, we try to find our own identity and often overidentify with pop heroes or movie stars. We become rabid Mick Jagger fans, we collect photos of David Bowie, we join fan clubs for this or that television idol. This is a particularly feminine attempt at the solution of the problem of identity: young boys do not have our capacity for loving identification, and so there are no female equivalents to —let's say—David Cassidy. This was true of our mothers too: there never was a female Frank Sinatra. Collecting photographs, concert programs, and LP records, we lose ourselves in being in love with someone whom everyone else loves too. For the moment, we find our identity by losing it; if nobody else screamed at a Sly concert, we would not scream ourselves. We do not want to be uniquely in love with him; it is our joy to submerge ourselves and our flickering sense of identity in that powerful mass that adores him, but whose sheer numbers give us power over him: *he must please us*.

In our fantasies, we go one step farther: the beloved idol, whose fate and fortune are made of enormous numbers, sees only one: us. Errol Flynn picks out

Katherine to dance with, among all the other beauties at the ball. Elvis "picks me out of the whole crowd to come to his hotel room," writes eighteen-year-old Jenny (who is a virgin), "and I end up going off to live with him. . . ." The star picks us out to love; he seats us beside him at his table, takes only us to his bed. Not only must we exist, but we must be beautiful, exciting, lovable over all other women. In these fantasies, the star gives us part of his magic and charisma. He shares the plentitude of love he gets from his fans with us. We grow rich on other women's envy; we are excited in ourselves by his fame. He is the sun, and we are the moon, shining beautifully in his reflected light.

All of which is enough—*plenty*—when we are in our teens. When we are women, these fantasies come to an end. We want to be seen in our own light. □

Jenny

I enjoyed your book, *My Secret Garden*. It's for, by, and about the female sex, and we need more books like that. I must admit that I was shocked at first by some of the fantasies—mine are never that explicit or far out. But perhaps they will become more so as I grow older. They've given me some great ideas, and I must admit that the pieces on animals fascinated me.

I am eighteen years old, and a virgin. Perhaps this is why my fantasies are so "mild" compared to the ones told in your first book. I fantasize going to a Hollywood party, and there meeting someone like Roddy McDowall or Gene Kelly (older men really turn me on). They immediately fall for me, and end up marrying me, or living together.

Sometimes I fantasize that I am at an Elvis concert, and he picks me out of the whole crowd to come up to his hotel room, and I end up going off to live with him at his home in Graceland.

Another fantasy I have concerns Mr. Spock from "Star

Trek." He is very unemotional and calm, but I could be the one to arouse him, and we'd end up making love, in a very dignified manner, however.

I also have the "classic" fantasies—being a kidnapped maiden, tied up in scanty rags, and just as the evil henchmen are about to attack me, the hero comes and whisks me off, but I assist him in fighting off the bad guys, with karate, etc. . . . No "weak damsel" for me!

I never plan on marrying, that's not the life for me—I want to be someone, go places, and see things. But I am also a Catholic, and that puts pressure on my moral beliefs. I would like to feel free to go to bed with anyone I like, but my religion forbids this. I don't want to be forever damned, but I don't wish to become a hermit, either. It's a bad scene.

Once again, thank you for the work you are doing. I hope it serves to show women that they're not alone in their dreams, and to encourage them to fantasize more. I truly believe that no man can ever have as great fantasies as we women have!

Veevee

I have read and reread your book, *My Secret Garden,* about a hundred times now, and I would like to make a contribution. Before I start, I want to tell you, that book is the greatest. What a relief when I learned that other girls fantasize too.

Now, about me. My name is Veevee. I am eighteen, I want to be a rock singer-costume designer, and I am very horny. I lost my virginity only last year to my boyfriend, who I am still dating. We have sex regularly, every weekend, even during my period. It's kind of messy, but he likes it, because he doesn't have to use a safe.

The men in my fantasies are neither black nor white, but Oriental. I find them extremely sexy, and I simply cannot warm up to any other kind of man (I'm not Oriental, though, myself). I detest hairy chests and faces

. . . pale hair, eyes, and skin are too milky to be erotic. I adore slim bodies, smooth golden skin, and cute asses, and Orientals have it all. Japanese are my favorites, and my boyfriend is a Japanese. I have also slept with a delicious Korean boy whom I met in another city recently. I haven't had a chance to lay out a Chinese yet, but I'm working on it.

The star of my fantasies *is* in fact a star, a Japanese rock singer superstar. He is incredibly gorgeous, with a mane of dark hair, great big black eyes, a complexion that a girl would envy, and a sensuous mouth just right for long deep kisses. And, wow, what a body! Not skinny at all, but smooth and well-muscled. I have some pictures of him wearing only shorts and track shoes, and I don't know how many times I have masturbated while looking at these photos. Anyway, I can fantasize him onstage, wearing a white leather outfit, with high boots and gloves, all studded with rhinestones. The pants and vest are really tight, and the vest is low cut. He is sleeveless, and his golden skin is gleaming with sweat under the lights. His hair is wild, and his eyes are flashing as he writhes and gyrates to the heavy throb of the music. Thousands of girls are screaming around him, but I watch him triumphantly, knowing that I am the woman who will possess that beautiful body, straining against the leather. Of all the women in the audience, only I can close my eyes and remember the exact shape of his cock—something no one else in the audience has ever seen, except tantalizingly when the excitement of his singing makes his erection show to the audience of screaming women through his tight trousers. Now he is taking his final bows, and I move off, out of the crowd, to grab a taxi to his apartment. As I walk through the crowd, nobody turns to look at me. They are all straining for a glimpse of him, but I have the secret power of knowing that if only they knew where I was going, and who I was soon going to be with, they would be clutching after me too.

Once in his apartment, I relax on his huge double bed.

It has satin sheets and a canopy with embroidered quilts. I sip a drink, until I hear the door open. He strides in and regards me for a moment through narrowed eyes. I can see that all that heavy music and dancing has had its effect, and I quiver with anticipation. I can feel the moisture begin between my legs. Without bothering to take anything off, he seizes me in his arms and kisses me firmly and urgently, meanwhile stripping off my clothes. My panties get snagged, and there is a satisfying sound of tearing, as he rips the cloth off my hips.

Now he removes his gloves and begins to caress my body, his golden hands moving from my breasts down to my belly, to my cunt (which I keep clean-shaven). He stands right in front of me, one arm around my neck, pulling me closer to him, the other hand down between my legs, his middle finger inside me, stirring up the juices as his tongue inside my mouth licks mine. I can hear myself sigh as I take a step with one foot to open my legs wider for him to put in two fingers.

His kisses become more insistent as they now begin to fall on my naked flesh lower and lower down, down, down, and his tongue in my hot cunt is just too much, and I heave and writhe in the most wonderful climax I have ever had—the cunt juices just flowing out of me and making a river down the crack of my ass.

This drives him wild, and he leaps on me and drives his long hard cock in so deep I moan with ecstasy. He is still wearing the leather vest, and I can see him thrusting and my legs wrapped around his ass in a mirror. He sees that I like looking at us in the mirror, and with a strong lunge of his cock, while he is still inside me, he pushes my ass around so that now we are parallel to the mirror, and I can actually see his long cock sliding in and out. I put my hand around it, as if to make my cunt longer and more firmly gripping. It excites him even more to be held by my hand and my cunt at the same time, and just as I slip my hand between his legs and shove a finger in his asshole, he shrieks as if he's being murdered. and he comes!

He is thoroughly exhausted by now, and I roll him on his back and gently undress him. I go to the washroom and clean myself up and fetch a cool towel to wipe him off with. I rub him with the towel on his back and chest, while he lies there watching me through half-closed eyes and smiling Then I massage his legs and back, and he sighs contentedly. I crawl back into bed with him, and we snuggle together and go to sleep in each other's arms.

This is one fantasy which I hope to make come true, but I don't know. . . . I intend to go to Japan this year. We'll see then. I get a real thrill out of pampering a guy and being pampered by him too. I like to be dominated somewhat. Because I am a big girl, I do most of the dominating in real life, but I'd like to take the passive role—in sex, anyway.

It was also great to find out other girls like to look at guys too. I enjoy supertight hiphugging pants with button flies on a guy with a pert, round ass and tapered thighs. I also like the curve between the shoulder and hip to be well-defined, and shirts to be unbuttoned at the neck. Tight high-waisted pants are great. I find boots very sexy. while shoes for some reason really make me cream my jeans. When my boyfirned wears his white shoes, it takes all my willpower not to take him then and there. White boots are superdynamite! I met a Chinese singer in a rock group who wore them, along with a tight jumpsuit unzipped almost to his navel. Zowie! I would have given my eyeteeth for just one round between the sheets with him.

Well, enough of what makes me horny. I hope you can use my fantasy. I know it is nothing fantastic, but when I am feeling low or nonsexy, all I have to do is imagine it, and I feel full of zip again. It is especially good to imagine it on nights when I am with my real boyfriend—it brings me to orgasm in ten seconds flat.

Katherine

My fantasies are nearly always about public figures—movie stars, baseball players, etc. I am twenty-two, pretty. single. in love twice, both times disasters, now cautious about men.

I have one fantasy wherein I am a fifteen-year-old girl named Marjorie. and Christopher Lee (the English actor) is my godfather. He is visiting my parents, and I somehow spirit him into the wooded area of our estate. I tell him I have a surprise for him, and he should turn his back to me. Soon I tell him to turn around, and he sees I am standing nude, smiling mischievously at him. He tries to think of a gentle let-down, but I throw myself at him, and he takes me there, in the middle of the woods.

Another fantasy is one where I seduce Basil Rathbone as Sherlock Holmes at 22B Baker St. In it, I am his twenty-year-old niece. Dr. Watson (Nigel Bruce) is amazed his aloof pal Holmes finally fell for someone.

I have another fantasy in which I am dancing at a ball; all the women are in flowing gowns and everyone is waltzing. My gown is so low-cut that my partner can look down and see my rosy nipples. Since it is Victorian times. I am a real virginal prude. My partner (let's call him Errol Flynn) takes me to a dark stairway outside the ballroom and pulls the top of my dress down. I object feebly as he massages my breasts. I get so aroused I can't fight it. and he lifts my long dress up and puts his fingers into me. The fear of being seen by the other guests adds to the excitement.

I have fantasies wherein a man fingers me under the tablecloth in a crowded restaurant.

Another one is that I am really drunk, too drunk to know what's going on, and I'm parked in a car with, oh, let's say Robert Taylor. He lays me across the front seat, lifts my dress, and pulls my panties down. Then he puts an empty wine bottle, thin neck first, of course, into me and moves it in and out really fast. I *writhe* in drunken ecstasy!

Well, those are a few of my most popular ones. I just LOVE those public figures! I often wonder how I'd react if I ever met one in the flesh; oh, I know some are already dead, but Christopher Lee, David Carradine ("Kung Fu"), Leonard Nimoy and William Shatner ("Star Trek"), and many of the N.Y. Mets, Nets, Jets, and Sets are still around. Sigh! I wonder what *their* wives fantasize about—or if they have to fantasize at all!

Muffie

I know ths will sound stupid, 'cause I'm not a silly teenage groupie, but rock singer Cat Stevens turns me on something fierce. I once stayed up until 3 A.M. watching a concert of his on television and masturbating myself senseless.

I fantasize that he and I are on a deserted beach laughing and running, naked. I trip and fall, and he rushes over to see if I'm all right. His hand on my naked back makes me burn, and with a moan, I roll over and pull him onto me, holding him gently, kissing his face and his eyes, his lips, and then burying my head in the soft hollow of his shoulder.

His caresses are gentle, like a thought, and his eyes are loving. Then without speaking, my legs open, and he enters me, pushing his cock against me easily, as if asking permission. Then we are fucking, and it seems like we are one with the sand, the sea, and the moon. When we finally come, it's graceful, unhurried. We fall asleep still entwined; when I awaken at dawn, he's gone, and I find a beautiful seashell in my hand, and it seems to be smiling at me.

I have really enjoyed being able to put the private me into words, so thank you. I am trying to get my friends to write you, but most are wrapped up in their garden clubs and dinners. Telling a fantasy to me and writing to you are worlds apart. Maybe one day they can be really free.

God bless you, Nancy. I'm glad someone cares enough to undertake understanding the *whole* woman.

Carina

I read your book and enjoyed it very much. Thank you for bringing out into the open that women think about sex more than some people realize. Here is a fantasy of mine for your new book.

First off, my name is Carina. I'm eighteen and live with my mother and two young brothers. My fantasy always takes place in the shower when I stand in a certain was so that the water hits me in the right spot of desire. In the fantasy, I'm washing in the shower and don't hear the doorbell ring. James Caan, the movie star, is at the door, and he walks right in (because he finds the door is accidentally unlocked). He's there because he's met a friend of mine who told him all about me. Well, he comes (I mean he pokes his head through the shower curtain) right into the shower, shedding his clothes and says: "Your friend was right. You are as marvelous as she said you were!" We make love while the water trickles over, around, and under our bodies. By this time, I have an orgasm and the fantasy ends.

I hope it is one that you can use.

☐ Though June is nineteen and married, she fantasizes about a girl friend she has known since she was thirteen. "In real life, as far as we got was to hold and kiss each other," she writes in lament about the children's sexual games they used to play in early adolescence. It seemed so easy then, so comforting to our loneliness, to see our friends as our other selves. We clung to each other for reassurance in young fear and bewilderment of our burgeoning sexuality. In exploring our friend's body, we explored our own.

This element of narcissistic identification seems clear in June's fantasy: she does not see her friend as a rival in the triangle she wants to set up with her own husband; she is not "the other woman"—she is an accomplice. Her fantasy reminds us of those days when doing anything was much more fun when we shared it with a girl friend . . . those early days when the true excitement of a date was not so much when we were with *him* but when we could describe it afterward to our friends.

One important point remains to be made about fantasies like June's: it is as common for women to have sexual fantasies about other women as it is rare for men to have fantasies about other men. The bugaboo of homosexual fear does not haunt our sex the way it does the other, but this does not mean that every woman who has a sexual fantasy about another woman is a lesbian. (The phrase "latent lesbian" has no meaning. We are all "latent"—it is imaginable for any human being to do something sexual with any other human being in the right time and circumstances.)

Some women who have fantasies about other women describe themselves as lesbians. Many women who have similar fantasies do not. You know yourself better than I do. Having a fantasy in your mind is a very far cry from meaning you have done something in actuality . . . or that you "really" want to do it. June has sexual fantasies about other women, but does not for one moment mention the idea that she might be a homosexual. Tina writes about her attraction to Barbara in terms that may well mean that in time she will enter a homosexual relationship. Scattered throughout this book are fantasies by other women who have erotic reveries about sex with other females . . . some letters are from women who have put this idea into practice. None of these sexual paths is better than any other, none is right or wrong. All that matters is how your sex life makes you feel. If you feel whole and happy, released and vital, it is nobody's business how you reach that goal. Some of the women concerned call themselves lesbians, others do not. What you call yourself is your business too.

In general, it can be said that sexual fantasies of other women can usually be traced back to feelings and emotions of babyhood, when our mother was our first love object. In time, as we grew up, we made the crossover to men—starting with father, who we took to be our first model for all men. But some leftover emotion about mother, some unconscious image of how she smelled, touched us, and gave us our first idea of love, is often still buried somewhere within us, just as there is a little bit of the child left over in every adult. □

June

I have just finished reading your book. I have really enjoyed it, and am glad someone has finally written about women's fantasies.

I have a few, but this is my favorite. This fantasy is always about a girl friend I've known since I was thirteen years old.

I've always wanted to make it with her. In real life, as far as we got was to hold and kiss each other. I have had women make love to me, but it's always turned me off. I know that (I'll call her Sue) Sue would be the only one that could turn me on.

I am nineteen years old and am married. I have told my husband before about my fantasy, but after I read your book, I got really excited and decided to really describe to him my fantasy and how I'd like him to be making it with the both of us. It really turned him on. We had the best time in bed than we've had in a long time.

We both hope someday our fantasy will come true. I

think then I would be the happiest. We live far from her now, but plan on moving back soon.

Well, thank you for the book you've written. I'm looking forward to your next book. I hope this can help you in some way.

Tina

I am thirty-seven years old and have been with my husband for fifteen years, the last ten of which I have known Barbara. My husband is sexually okay, but not passionate—his value as a husband is based on other qualities. My strongest emotional need has been to be able to be open, to share all my thoughts and feelings (including sexual fantasies). I have done this not with my husband but with Barbara. She has also shared more deeply with me than with anyone else until recently, when someone new entered her life.

I have had sexual fantasies about her and other women for as long as I can remember having sexual feelings at all. The reason I am writing to you now is because of "the change" in me—none of the fantasies in your book seem to cover that part of me.

As time has gone by, the outward sexuality between Barb and me has grown from no touching at all to spontaneous kisses and embraces and back rubs that take me close to orgasm. (I think the next time I will ask if she minds for me to masturbate in her presence. I will have to think about this for a while since we live in separate cities, and our direct contact is only once or twice a year.)

Until last year, Barbara said that she wasn't sexually attracted to women. Now she is living in a lesbian relationship. You can imagine the mixture of joy for her and pain I felt for myself when that happened. Until the beginning of that relationship, my fantasies about women had always been about Barbara. I would imagine her saying "Yes, I do have sexual feelings for you," and going down on me, hugging, kissing, etc. Once I imagined Barb walking in while I was masturbating and sitting down beside me and holding my left hand. Last winter, I visited with her and her lover and had the deepest back rub yet. The whole time she was much more open and affectionate than ever before, but still clear that I wasn't to be her bedmate. The next night, we three women did pot together (my first time). Eventually, they went to the bedroom, and I lay down on the couch. I felt like I was with them, part of their sex. And then suddenly switching from explicit masturbatory images, I was talking to Barb, sharing with her words of love and deep feelings, some of it even admissions of jealousy. But even though what I was telling her was not all positive feelings, I could sense Barb's understanding and love. Her nonsexual but deep love for me wanting me to feel good and enhancing my sexual intensity. Since then I have often incorporated this sense of feeling close with a woman, feeling her love with my masturbation. I told Barbara the next day, and she felt it was a beautiful thing. I shared all the feelings too that I had verbalized in the fantasy when I had imagined the two of them making love in the other room, and she understood all of that too. I suppose you might not call this a sexual fantasy, but it turns me on deepest of all when I masturbate to imagine how deeply a woman (Barb) understands me, accepts and loves me. Sometimes I try to incorporate this feeling into my time with my husband (but I do feel guilty thinking of someone else when I am with him). I have since last winter slept with three women. One of them touched my deepest feelings along with my body. I fantasize about her both ways at once—the feelings that we share, plus the memories of our sex. Love and sex together can be a very powerful stimulant.

I see myself as bisexual, by the way, and have been working within my religious denomination to spread understanding of homosexuality and bisexuality. I initiated a consideration of these issues in Barb's state last summer, before it was an active concern to her. This summer, she stood where I had stood with the others and carried it through, while I stayed in my own territory. I am more than pleased by the feelings of togetherness and sisterhood I get from these activities.

I told one of my lovers about this kind of fantasy, and she tried it and really liked it. I hope I have explained it well enough so that you understand. It's the strength of emotional intensity and general closeness that heightens sexual feelings. Also, one of my explicit fantasies wasn't mentioned until now. I'll say it quickly before I lose my nerve. I am drinking breast milk and eventually floating in it, and as I approach climax, I feel myself drowning.

□ Toby's first fantasy, like most in this chapter, stems from a time in her life when she was not yet ready for sex. She was fifteen, she writes, when she began to fantasize about the man who lived next door. He was "about forty-five, with sexy gray hair (sophisticated-looking)."

Ah, these sophisticated-looking, gray-haired older devils! How often they populate the erotic reveries of women young enough to be their daughters. The ambiguous mystery they bring with them, of having slept in many beds, surrounds them with an almost mystic, golden haze of romance. Sexual but fatherly at the same time, the older man promises to guide us safely into our sexual life, initiating us with his great skill, forgiving us in his wisdom by joining us in the forbidden act. □

Toby

I'm eighteen, white, single, and reasonably sexually liberated, surrounded by people who frown upon sex. Right now, I'm having an affair with a guy called Lou, who is twenty-six. His divorce comes through in about one month. He's really fantastic!

My first fantasy was of a man who lived next door to us. At our summer cottage. I was fifteen at the time. He's about forty-five, with sexy gray hair (sophisticated-looking).

My parents have one cottage while I have my own.

At about one in the morning, a knock would come at the door and V., the man next door, who had kids older than I, would come in and immediately we'd be locked in a mad embrace. He was the best married man around.

Whispering gentle words, we'd fall on the bed and make love. He's gentle and I get horny thinking about him. We'll screw and talk until five A.M., when he returns home and leaves me with memories.

Another fantasy I have is having a huge dog (German shepherd) make love to me (doggie-style, of course). I would be held down, and the dog would be forced to sniff between my legs and lick me out. Then he'd put his hard, moist penis inside me, and we'd rock on to heaven.

Just the thought of his big nose probing between my legs excites me.

Nothing really excites me as the thought of making love to two men. Both of whom are familiar to me.

One to perform cunnilingus on me while the other (after the first) can screw me.

While on a train, Lou and I made love on the seats of our car. It was dark, at night, so no one really saw us (I hope). The seats across from me were vacant, but there were people ahead and behind me. We played with each other until that crucial moment came. He pulled down his pants and put a blanket over him. I had on a dress with no pants, so I just hopped on his knee, and when he put his huge prick inside me, along with the movement of the train, it was heaven. It was good! I experienced my first real orgasm with him.

We fucked for about two hours, all the way to Boston, where we had an engagement to play the next day.

I'll often fantasize that again he's home, and I can screw him again and again and again.

Everytime I see a guy in tight pants . . . look out! I could just grab him and wow!!

You seem like a fantastic lady, and I hope we could meet sometime.

Penny

When I first became aware of my sexual fantasies, I was in my early teens. They used to threaten me sometimes, particularly the ones involving other women. I have not gotten to the point even today where I can, or want to discuss them with my husband, even though my best friend and I swap fantasies. Our latest mutual fantasy is telling our men that we're going to Memphis for a weekend shopping spree, but actually going there to get fucked. As you can see, I have come a long way with my fantasies, and can now enjoy them. In fact, I don't like to read *My Secret Garden* while I'm at work, because it gets me too turned on, and that's not a state I want to be in at the office.

One of my favorite fantasies when I was a kid was walking along the superhighway near the school I went to. The people weren't in cars—I would imagine them moving together in small clumps or groups, but walking. As I moved into the left lane to pass a slow-moving family, I had to turn sideways. I passed close by a man with a hard-on. I smiled and said mm—mm—mm . . . as in mm—mm—good. He took my arm and tried to get me to go with him. I smiled sheepishly and answered that I really couldn't, because I was too young and inexperienced. He tried to convince me again, and I said, why not. We got out at the next exit. I had no pants on. We were sitting near the school. Someone (I think the hard-on man) was twiddling my clit. It felt good. Then I was in a room. I decided I had to get out. So I sheepishly asked him if I could please have my pants back. He gave them to me, and I hurriedly left the room. There was snow on the ground; then the man was after me. All of a sudden, I saw a train arriving. I yelled out, "Thank God for the Southern Pacific!"

That was the end of that particular one. One of the first fantasies I can remember in my whole life was a man lying down. I opened his zipper—I thrust my hand inside his pants, but into pitch blackness. At that time, I had never seen a cock.

A couple of years ago, when I went through the phase I described of having fantasies about other women, my sexual images were very exotic. I would imagine myself grabbing Miss America's tit, watching a pregnant lady undress. Many times, I have had dreams about being bare-chested in public, in which I usually tried to cover myself. Recently, I had celebrity week. One night, I was part of the *M.A.S.H.* unit, and Alan Alda was after me. The next night, Frank Langella (*Diary of a Mad Housewife, Twelve Chairs*) was fucking me and said, "The only problem is that I have a small dick. So you will have to flex your muscle." I remember in my dream feeling my vagina tighten and loosen, tighten and loosen.

If you like, I can ask the friend I swap fantasies with to send you hers. I hope I have been of some help.

Cecillia

I love you, I love you, I love you!!!!
Your book was sensational and quite a turn on at times—a turn off at others, but always devilishly good fun. I'd love very much to submit a fantasy or two of my own. I'm seventeen, and have fantasized (in one form or another) as long as I can remember.

My favorite (current favorite, that is) concerns this boy I went out with several times (but unfortunately never slept with). This was while I was still a virgin—but should I run into him again, am sure I could get things to happen!! The fantasy starts that we're in his bedroom, alone together, and I walk over to him and just start to kiss him quite passionately while I unzip his fly. I take his huge throbbing cock into my hands and start caressing, fondling it, etc. He slips his trembling hands up my sweater and starts to massage my breasts. He has to unzip my fly and slips his hand right on my dripping pussy and sticks a few fingers up my cunt.

We both undress each other (I stop while pulling off his pants to fellate him). He lays me on his bed, props my legs up and open, and his full red lips unite with my red cunt and *Zowie!* I pull his head into me, and that tongue of his licks the hell out of me. We have intercourse and both end up quite satisfied.

My next one concerns a girl friend of mine. I decide to sleep over her house, so we smoke some grass and are feeling rather free with one another. We decide to take a shower together, and that's when the fun begins. We offer to wash one another's backs and naturally that's not all we wash of one another. We get into her bedroom and first I towel her off, then she does me; she has me sit on the edge of her bed so that she can dry my feet and legs She starts feeling my thighs and starts to kiss and lick them. She opens my legs wide and starts to lick, suck, and kiss my cunt. She works her way all over me, and we end up 69ing it all night.

I've told my lover these, and he enjoys them also.

I too am an avid crotch- and fanny-watcher. I always enjoy visually undressing men and imagining screwing with them. Can't wait for your next book. Much love to you.

Isabel

I just finished reading your book called *My Secret Garden*, and I liked it very much. I especially liked it because it made me feel better about myself. I think about sex a lot, and I fantasize about sex so much that I was beginning to think that I was perverted. It makes me feel better to know that other women fantasize about sex just as I do. I am going to be a sophomore in college this next school year, but I am home for the summer right now. I want to tell you about my fantasies, but I must keep this letter anonymous, because I live in a very small town, and I do not want anyone here to find out about me. As I said, I have a lot of sexual fantasies, and I would like to tell you about some of them. Although I have sexual fantasies almost anytime, I have my most developed sexual fantasies when I masturbate. I think I masturbate more than most girls. Almost every night before I go to sleep, I masturbate, and I often masturbate at other times during the day when I am aroused and can be alone for a while. Masturbation is the only kind of sexual activity I have ever had. Although people say I have a pretty face, I am overweight. Being overweight makes it difficult for me to get dates with boys, so I have had only a few dates with boys in my whole life. To be honest, I am a little afraid of boys. I am afraid I might be frigid if I ever did have sex with a boy. That's enough about me though. I had better tell you about my fantasies.

I think I am the female equivalent of a "peeping Tom." In my sexual fantasies, I almost always imagine myself secretly watching other persons engaged in sexual activities. One of my favorites is to imagine an attractive boy undressing while I am secretly watching him. I have never seen a boy undressed, so I am not sure if what I imagine is completely accurate. I am aroused by the thought of seeing a boy's sexual organs, but the thought of actually touching them kind of scares me. They kind of attract and repulse me at the same time. When I have this fantasy, I also like to imagine this boy masturbating himself after he undresses. I am not sure how boys really do masturbate themselves, but in my fantasies they do it several ways. My favorite right now is to imagine a boy lying facedown on his bed and moving his hips up and down so that his penis rubs against the sheets. I like to imagine that when he ejaculates he calls out my name as though he has been fantasizing about me.

Another of my fantasies is to imagine a couple having sex while I secretly watch. The couples are usually persons I know personally; when one of my girl friends gets married, I like to lie in my bed on her wedding night and try to imagine what she and her new husband may be doing. I imagine that I am there secretly watching when she sees her husband undress for the first time and when she undresses while her husband watches. The thought of undressing in front of a boy scares me, but it arouses me too. After fantasizing about one of my girl friends and her new husband undressing, I imagine that I am secretly watching them when they have sex for the first time. Unless I know otherwise for sure, I imagine that she is a virgin. Her husband's penis is very large, and she cries out with pain when he pushes it into her for the first time. It hurts so much that she starts crying, but in a few minutes, it starts to feel good to her. This, too, is a part of sex that scares me, but also arouses me.

Besides newlyweds, I fantasize about other couples I know too, both married and unmarried. I think about what they probably do when they have sex. I like to try and imagine all the things they might do when they are having sex together. In my mind, I try to picture them having sex. One of my favorite things is to imagine them having oral sex. Mostly, I try to picture whatever girl I am fantasizing about sucking on her partner's penis. The idea of doing that to a boy repulses me, and yet it fascinates me too. I sometimes imagine that he ejaculates in her mouth and that she swallows it. Thinking about that arouses me very much, but I do not think that I would ever really do that myself. I also like to picture in my mind couples masturbating each other, and I get very aroused when I try to picture the boy sucking on the girl's nipples.

Most of my sexual fantasies are of the types I have already described, but I do have a few other kinds of sexual fantasies sometimes. Almost everytime I see a good-looking boy, I try to imagine what he looks like with his clothes off. When I do this, I kind of play a game.

I try to guess the size and shape of his sexual organs, although having never seen a boy with his clothes off, I am not too sure what his sexual organs ought to look like. Once I saw a boy whose pants were bulging as though his penis were erect, and it arouses me when I think about how he looked. I really wish that there were a magazine for women that showed photographs of good-looking men with all their clothes off. Another fantasy that I have had a few times concerns two girls I know at college. They have an apartment together, and I found out from some of my friends that they are lesbians. Sometimes when I masturbate, I try to imagine that I am secretly watching when these two girls are having sex together. It worries me, but I do get very aroused when I think about them having sex. Sometimes I get aroused thinking about some very feminine and slim girl with all her clothes off, and occasionally I fantasize about secretly watching a girl like that undress and then masturbate. Sometimes I think that I would be less afraid of having sex with another girl than I would of having sex with a boy.

In almost all my sexual fantasies, I am just a secret observer of other persons' sexual activities, but in a very small number of fantasies, I do play other parts. Most of these fantasies have a similar format. I imagine that I am trapped and am forced to have sex with a good-looking boy. I will give you an example of one of these fantasies. I imagine that I and a good-looking boy, who otherwise would pay no attention to me, are snowbound alone together in a mountain cabin together or some other place like that. We have food and logs for the fire in the fireplace, so we are comfortable. When night comes, we prepare to sleep in separate rooms, but when I begin undressing, he bursts into my room. He already has all his clothes off, and he forceably removes the rest of my clothing. When he sees me with my clothes off, he gets even more excited, and his penis becomes erect. It is very firm and very large, and I am scared by the sight of it. He forces me down on my back on the bed and gets on

101

top of me. Right away he starts trying to push his penis into me. It hurts so much that I start crying, but he just keeps pushing his penis into me. After several minutes of that, it begins to feel good. He keeps moving his penis in and out of me for about ten or fifteen minutes, and then he ejaculates. While he is ejaculating, he tells me how good it feels to have sex with me. Afterward, we lie in bed together, and he is very affectionate to me. In fantasies like this one, I imagine that having sex feels very good, but I do not have an orgasm in them. I do not have this kind of fantasy very often though. I probably only have it about once or twice a month. I have to be in just the right mood for this kind or else they make me feel bad instead of good.

The first specifically sexual fantasy that I ever had occurred when I was thirteen, and my oldest sister got married (I only have sisters and no brothers). At that time, I asked my mother about marriage and having babies, and she told me about sex. Soon after that, I began to masturbate, and when I did, I would fantasize about being able to secretly watch while my sister and her new husband were having sex together. Maybe because it was the first kind of sexual fantasy I had, this kind of fantasy is just about my favorite of all. I get extremely aroused when I try to picture what a newly married couple I know are doing on their wedding night or on their honeymoon. Second to this kind of fantasy are those in which I imagine that I am secretly watching while a good-looking boy takes off all his clothes and then masturbates. I would MUCH RATHER imagine watching this than to actually have sex with a boy.

I hope that what I have told you about my sexual fantasies will help your continuing research. I can hardly wait to read the results of this additional research. I lent my copy of your book to a friend of mine, and she, too, likes it very much. Maybe she will write to you too. I might even write to you again if I think of more to tell you about.

CHAPTER THREE

LOOKING

☐ Until very recently, it was a cliché even in the medical profession that women were not turned on by reading pornography. When I began researching *My Secret Garden*, one doctor after another told me that women are *unable* to become aroused through the same kind of visual stimuli that moved men. "A woman does not look at sex as a kind of simple, physical proposition the way men can," went the usual explanation. "Pornographic books or photos leave all emotion out of sex, but unless a woman can see sex in an emotional context, she just isn't interested."

This may have sounded reasonable enough; on the whole, it is fairly true of the way women lead their lives. The only problem with the explanation is that it does not account for, or even acknowledge, *female lust.*

It did not help explain to me why. I would always find my eyes riveted to attention when I passed a man on the street who had a noticeable bulge in his trousers . . . why, when I went to see *The Changing Room*, a play in which at least a dozen naked men come on stage at one time, it was all I could do to keep my head from swiveling from side to side. I had never seen so many naked cocks presented for my inspection at one time, and although I felt no emotion for any of the actors involved, it was one of the most exciting evenings I had ever spent in a theater.

Was I some kind of freak? I wondered. I had nothing to compare myself to, no role-models whose footsteps I could safely walk in. I had no cultural okay to give sanction to my prurient interest, the way men have for theirs. If a man likes to go to burlesque shows and pins photos of naked women on his wall, it shows he is one hell of a lusty guy. There is even a society based in San Diego made up of young studs who proudly label themselves "International Girl Watchers." But we are only supposed to collect photos of couples walking hand in hand in the moonlight. The whole business seemed unfair to me—worse, it offended my sense of logic and symmetry. There must be a reverse to the coin, even if I had never heard it discussed, even if no doctor would agree with me. I remember talking to a friend's young daughter not too long ago about her experiences at the beach. "Men have these funny bulges in the front of their bathing suits," the girl said, "but you're not supposed to notice them. How do you do that?"

How indeed? I get furious when I hear men and women alike say that the naked male isn't as interesting or beautiful as the naked female. Why? Why should tits be any more beautiful than a man's buttocks or cock? I believe it is men themselves who've set up the idea that their naked bodies are ugly—or at least, too trivial or unimportant to look at, unless they have an errection! If I am right, then it is also men themselves who will have to help both sexes get over this absurd prejudice. Men are going to have to accept their own naked bodies as aesthetically satisfying, and not merely sexually useful; they will have to learn to lie back and enjoy allowing a woman to look at them. Once men can get away from the idea that they are not worth looking at if they don't have a giant, erect cock, they will be liberated from an enormous amount of their castration anxieties. They will be freed from the notion that they are either a giant penis or they are "nothing." They can be men, instead of perpetual fucking machines.

To see a naked man from the rear is a sight that takes my breath away—the awesome shape of power as the shoulders drop away into narrow hips, the hard, muscle-bunched look of an athlete's ass. . . . There are lines in the male body that have never been mentioned, aesthetics of masculine anatomy women will soon be writing poetry about . . . *if* we can give ourselves permission to look.

Unlike men, women have been trained from birth to be exhibitionists. Fashion is busily revealing one aspect of our anatomy this year, hiding it the next. Who more than a woman feels more deeply in her bones the erotic power of what the eye can see? It is obvious to me that both sexes must be equally stimulated by reading and seeing sexual sights, but that women—"ladies"—have been culturally conditioned to deny it, even to themselves. *Both* sexes respond to natural things like sunshine, furry animals, the feeling of speed, the sound of music—why should there be this great divide in what turns on the individual sexes? If both women and men like sex, both must like it in all its manifestations, even the most fleeting. After I had written in *My Secret Garden* that I was "an inveterate crotch-watcher," woman after woman has taken me aside to tell me, with a relieved laugh, that she was too. (You will also find mention of the pleasures of fantasizing what goes on under a man's tight-fitting pants in many of the letters in this book.)

Roxanne too sends evidence that I'm not alone in getting an erotic charge out of things I see. Her letter contains eleven different fantasies, all of which involve looking and being looked at.

But her letter ends on a sad note, I feel—one that does much to explain why women are so afraid to confess their excitement at seeing something sexual. ". . . I must stop now," Roxanne concludes, "as my husband is coming home. He's great but rather traditional, so I don't want him to see all this." Instead of seeing women's sexual response to things they see or read as one more erotic avenue to explore together, too many men see it as a threat, a sign of raging sexuality that they are afraid they may not be able to satisfy. "My ex-husband would rather think of me as frigid," a friend recently said to me, "than think maybe I wasn't getting enough." □

Roxanne

I have a number of favorite fantasies—I say favorite because if I described all of my fantasies I'd be able to write a book myself. So anyway, as my vaginal juices start proliferating, here goes:

Fantasy 1: There is a pornographic book and magazine store fairly near where I live. The magazines are especially great, with *all types* of pictures and advice, including how guys can best fuck guys, and so forth. Anyway, I see myself going in there with some type of revealing clothing on and definitely NO underwear of any kind. Whatever the top material is, my nipples will be clearly visible, and the bottom part will be some sort of skirt-dress. I go in and start paging through some magazines when I accidently on purpose drop one. I bend over to pick it up, thus revealing my ass and cunt in all their glory. The young male proprietor naturally is watching me all along, and he has all he can do to contain himself. Sometimes he'll rush over and before I even get a chance to get up, he sticks his enormous prick in me—in my asshole, in my cunt—no matter—and pumps to our hearts' delight.

Sometimes he won't approach me, so I'll take a few magazines to him to purchase and say, "Boy, I'll bet you get horny working in a place like this," or "You should have a back room where horny females like me can get some fucking when they need it—like right now." He looks at me with lust and tells me they do have such a room! He directs me and in I go with my throbbing body. What should be in there but three gorgeous guys, and I direct the show. Wow—have you ever had all three holes fucked simultaneously?

Another great feeling is to be held by two guys and raised up and down on a third guy's prick—first slowly and then with progressive speed.

After all this, I still want more variety. I take one guy

into the adjoining shower with me and ask him to pee on me—yes—pee on my boobs and tummy and cunt. That's exciting! After that, I bend over on all fours and tell him to "stick it up my ass," which he obligingly does.

This particular fantasy usually ends about here. This very morning, I went to the bookstore to act this out (at least in the initial stages) only to find out they had gone out of business. Would you believe that? And I was *ready!* All I had on was a white peasant blouse off-the-shoulders and a short peasant type skirt—no undies! If I had bent over or if a good wind had come along, I either would've been arrested or raped—maybe both. I sure was disappointed and frustrated! I went home and masturbated with an artificial banana, which, believe me, was no substitute for a cock (or cocks).

Fantasy 2: I have tremendous exhibitionist urges—like the bending over previously described. I get a lot of these ideas from looking at magazine photos. I'd LOVE to perform a strip act which culminated in fucking the whole damn male audience. I'd like to masturbate manually or with cucumbers or whatever on stage and drive men to distraction.

Fantasy 3: I'd like to be casually dressed in some public place as a department store with my button-down-the-front blouse open just far enough to let a boob show from the side for the benefit of male passersby. Occasionally, someone grabs it and starts tearing my clothes off from lust.

Fantasy 4: Here's something I actually did a few weeks ago. I again had on no underwear, and I parked my car in a parking lot next to a tall building where construction was being carried out. There were workmen a few floors above me, so I decided to give them a treat. . . . I pulled my skirt up (in the car) and began to masturbate with my finger. After a few minutes, I had quite an appreciative audience. I would've liked screwing one or more of them, but time pressures didn't allow. Alas!

Fantasy 5: I'd love to be seeing a porno film in a theater—I can feel and see myself getting hot and wet because the film is really turning me on. All of a sudden, I feel a strange hand on my thigh slowly heading for my black tiny bikini panties. The hand reaches its mark and finds me wet and ready. To avoid creating too much of a disturbance, I remove the panties, and he opens his fly. I move over and sit on his lap thereby causing his twelve-inch-long sex tool to go easily and smoothly into my burning sex hole—up and down I go till we exhaust ourselves in climax. Then we part and he moves to a different location in the darkened theater. I've never seen his face—it wasn't necessary.

I just now stuck my finger up my twat as I'm writing this—my god—I don't even feel human—just one whole sex machine.

Fantasy 6: At other times, I see myself as a teacher of middle-to-late teen years boys. They don't especially turn me on, but I'd like to sit on the desk with my legs apart and turn THEM on by letting them see my sex organs "accidentally." Sometimes, a cooperative fellow teacher (male) comes into the room, and we demonstrate to them "proper" oral lovemaking. He undresses me slowly and completely, and I again sit on the desk—now completely naked. He asks me to sit with my legs apart so the whole class can see my cunt and asshole. *He* spreads my labia part and describes my female anatomy to the class. While he's touching and describing, I'm going crazy and am moving my body about in wild abandon. The boys at their desks are one-by-one opening their flies to let their cocks escape. Here and there, I see a fountain of semen exploding. My fellow teacher now goes down on me by titillating my clitoris with his tongue. He goes down slowly until his tongue slips into my vagina, and his finger is up my ass. I'm still on the desk. By now, boys are fucking boys and several are clawing at me—sucking my nipples and trying to move the teacher out of the way so they can get at me. This goes on and on. . . .

Fantasy 7: I really get turned on by looking at naked men in *Playgirl*. While looking, I sometimes imagine myself at home with minimal revealing clothing on—maybe a see-through shortie nightgown. I've been looking at myself in the full-length mirror in the bedroom and admiring my body. In front of the mirror, I've been executing some bumps and grinds in various stages of partial disrobing. I've also been watching myself masturbate. but this never really satisfies me, so I'm in one hell of a bad way when there's a knock on the front door. I go to the living room, peek through the blinds, and see a deliveryman with a package for me. By this time, he's really banging on the door, so I figure, "Oh, shit, if he's in such a hurry, I'll just open up." And open up I do—both the door and myself. When I open the door, he asks me to sign for the package; as I am signing, he is looking. When I finish signing, it is my turn to look—at his crotch. Needless to say, it is really bulging! He is standing slightly inside the door, so as I reach to close it behind him, my nipples brush his bare arm. That's all he needs. He grabs me, lifts me up, and carries me over to a living room chair, where he places me on the chair with one of my legs over each arm of the chair, thus leaving me slightly suspended and with my genitals completely exposed. He pulls up my nightgown over my head and leaves me with nothing on. I am so excited I can feel the juices coming out of me. He whips out of his pocket an artificial cock and sticks it in me—up and down it goes till I come and come and come. Then he picks me up and puts me on the floor and fucks me till I'm delirious. While this is going on, my dog enters the living room and starts sniffing and whining, and his prick starts popping out. He doesn't have a chance, though. because my deliveryman is delivering too good for me to pay any attention to my dog . . . maybe some other time.

Fantasy 8: I'd also like to find a guy who would like to lie down in the bathtub with me straddling him and let me pee all over him.

Fantasy 9: I occasionally visualize myself walking

into a college fraternity and announcing my availability for ANYONE who's there and ready.

Fantasy 10: I'm a patron in a strip-bar. The girl on stage is doing her thing and has nothing on but a G-string. I'm there alone, and the room is filled with men who are all excited from watching the stripper. Strippers excite me too—but I want a MAN to satisfy me. One approaches me, sits next to me, and puts his hand under my skirt. In a very short time, he's got four fingers in my hole, and I don't give a damn who's watching. Pretty soon, all eyes are on us. I'm laid out in the booth, and he's undressing. He gets on top of me, and then me on him; when I'm on top of him, my boobs are bouncing like crazy, and pretty soon I feel another prick going up my ass. We're all keeping time to the music. The stripper is still dancing, and she takes her G-string off and starts masturbating herself with a candle from one of the tables. People are applauding, yelling, and cussing, and the music gets louder and louder. It feels so good—it just never ends.

Fantasy 11: I love to pose for porno pictures in real life . . . not professionally—just for my lovers. God, that's exciting. I'll pose in ANY way regardless. You name it—I'll do it. I love to later look at the pictures and get excited all over again. Once, a guy and myself took a picture in a mirror of me sucking his cock—to look at that later was absolutely fascinating and thrilling.

I walk around most of the time in a horny condition. Sometimes I can't even concentrate, and that's bad because I'm a college-educated professional person. . . . I won't say what profession, because I can't risk identification in any way.

Well, there are more, but I must stop now as my husband is coming home. He's great but rather traditional, so I don't want him to see all this.

I'm anxious to read your second book—hope you can use some of this in it.

☐ A few years ago, I used to write frequently for *Cosmopolitan* magazine. I remember talking one day to Helen Gurley Brown. She was thinking of doing something very daring: she wanted to run a nude male centerfold. She wanted my help in finding the right man. I happily fell to thinking of who this Mr. Right could be, summoning up at least a dozen from my own fantasies. Helen was very anxious about the project: she was worried that it might turn off many women unless it was done in good taste. She had cause for her concern: it had never been done before in any woman's magazine published in America. What Helen didn't realize was that the women in her audience were more than ready for her experiment.

I had earlier discovered in my own research for *My Secret Garden* that the best way to relax women's anxiety about talking honestly about their erotic ideas was to tell them about my own behavior first. This gave them a role-model, someone they could identify with, and the feeling they were not alone in discussing any sexual area. Therefore, in the hundreds of questionnaires I circulated for *Garden,* I described myself as an "avid crotch-watcher," and asked if the reader was one too. That question never failed to get a response. Most women wrote that they were crotch-watchers too, others said they loved seeing "men's bottoms," "examining their pants to see which leg it hung down in," or just plain "looking." Sharon says, "I find myself many times looking at the crotches of men's pants, just as I sometimes find men gazing at my breasts!" "I've always been an inveterate crotch-watcher," Molly writes. "I love it when I see some guy with a partial erection. I am delighted to find I'm not alone."

The response I was getting (in a small way) to my questionnaire was multiplied a thousand times by the reaction to that first photo of the naked Burt Reynolds in *Cosmo.* If, for her own reasons, Helen Brown decided not to continue nude male photos as a regular feature, she nevertheless did found an entire industry. There are now several women's magazines that feature pages of naked men with ever-increasing variety and size of genitalia for the leisurely inspection of the women of America—many of whom had never before seen these mysterious parts of male anatomy up close and in living color.

If much of this photographic effort is still in bad taste—or more to the point, not to your taste—here are several reasons to explain it. One is that I don't think that these new magazines have figured out how to photograph the naked male in the way women would like to see a man. Perhaps the big clue to this is that the magazines in question are owned and published by men, or have male art directors. Therefore, the naked men are depicted in the way these men feel women would respond: the naked football player, hairy actor, or model is shown in all his muscular beauty alongside a stallion with flaring nostrils and a sexual organ rivaled only by the size of the model's . . . or else there is the inevitable Maserati or Ferrari vroom-vrooming alongside. The art director could not believe those poor women out there would "get it" unless the photo were power-packed with male phallic symbols. The man alone wasn't enough . . . these other men thought.

These new magazines have been grinding out male pinups now for a couple of years. Because I am all in favor of it, and only regret that they don't do it better, I am pleased to see that they are learning to drop the horses, cars, and other barbed-wire masculinity props. They must have begun to listen to the women "out there" instead of to the anxious noises in their own heads: a woman does not need any symbols to help her recognize that the naked penis she is looking at belongs to a man.

Another and still on-going misconception about what women enjoy in looking at naked men is the belief that if the penis isn't a foot long, no woman could be bothered. Once again, the question must be asked: Are the men who hold these fixed ideas getting them from their audience, or is it a response to their own, inner anxiety?

The idea that size is everything is the very turning point in the new Mel Brooks film, *The Young Frankenstein*. In this movie, the frigid, manipulative young woman has no qualms about brushing off her curly-haired lover, but is brought to orgasm and "womanhood" by the immensity of the monster's monstrous cock. At the point in the film where her eyes rivet on the gigantic tool approaching her maidenhead, her face registers fear and horror, but in the ensuing moment of penetration her voice reaches a relieved, resounding high C of song and exuberance. The audience breaks up with laughter; everybody gets the joke. But it's no joke in real life.

One of men's greatest sexual hang-ups concerns the size of their cock. They *really* believe that size is everything; psychiatrists do a lot of business treating patients with terrible complexes about the sexual inadequacy of their penis size. ("It's only seven inches, Doctor.") What hasn't come across to the people who create these films and centerfolds is that while women in this book, or in jokes among themselves, may go on about this or that "huge," "gigantic," or "monster" cock, the entire idea must be taken as a metaphor for the pleasure they desire . . . size is the purely symbolic measure of their exuberant approach to the joys of sex. What woman wants to be ripped open in real life by an enormous penis, jammed and made sore by some tremendous cock?

Women's insistence on size in their conversation or fantasies is merely the "handle" on which to hang their dreams. It is their cry for more sexual pleasure, for a larger, more intense experience—not a larger tool. I have heard very few women deplore the small size of their lover. As any doctor or experienced woman can tell you, it's not the quantity but the quality of the cock, the expertise of the lover.

This male preoccupation with, and fear about, his own inadequacy has so far bred (for me) a disappointing overindulgence in centerfold photos of men with penises so big and swollen there is no room for imagination. While Jackie writes that she is turned on by the intensely masochistic, but very well-written novel, *The Story of O*, and by other things she reads and sees, she finds no stimulation in "dirty movies," because they are "unimaginative and tasteless." To any man who says, "But what woman wants to see a limp cock?" I can only answer—"Who better than a woman knows what can be made of a limp cock?"

Give us something real to work with. I am all for photos of naked men being made available to us in women's magazines. I wish I'd had them when I was growing up. Why should men's genitalia be a mystery? But these magazines' success in the long run, is going to depend upon the development of an audience of women who have learned how to respond to the sight of naked men in films, photos, and all media. When women relax enough, and allow their own genuine emotions and reactions to enter their consciousness . . . when they feel free enough to play with the emotions aroused within themselves at the sight of these beautiful naked men . . . when they have learned "to look" and be honestly receptive . . . the message will get back to the industry, *and the industry will learn sophistication from its audience:* women enjoying looking; this is what they like to look at.

Any new industry takes time for supply and demand to get together, especially in an area so sensitive and taboo as women unashamedly looking and enjoying the sight of naked men. I hope we get enough time, that the art of photographing male nudes progresses so that it can command a genuine mass audience, month after month, year after year. I hope the opportunity for women to see and enjoy the male nude is not just a passing fad. It answers a very real sexual need among women . . . and anything that does can only reflect beneficially on men.

I believe it will happen. If nothing else, we are a tyrannically commercial country. Industry has long known it could use feminine sex appeal to sell men anything from convertibles to mutual funds. Once it becomes clear that male sex appeal can work the same salesmanship wonders with women, the state of the art will move ahead with the speed of a cash register ringing up a dollar sign. I am not applauding mindless materialism. I am merely saying that one of the serendipitous by-products of the inevitable growth in the use of male sex appeal by the advertising industry is that it will at last give women social sanction to enjoy being the looker-at last—and not always and only the looked-at. □

Sharon

I have just finished reading your book, *My Secret Garden*. I would like to say thanks for writing such a book. I felt I should write and tell you my fantasies (sexual). But first, I think it is necessary for you to know a little about me. I am a single, nineteen-year-old sophomore in college. I attend a small junior college here in my hometown. Because the town is so small, everybody, especially the young people, know practically everyone else. My parents are pretty uptight about sex. My mother only told me the basics about menstruation and all that, which I already knew when she finally told me. My father never told me anything! I have two brothers whom I have helped bathe, and I used to baby-sit for four boys a lot, so I've known for a long time what a penis looked like. The penis has always intrigued me, so when I became able to read such advanced material, I did just that. Reading books and magazines is the way I've learned about sex and the male and female bodies. I masturbate occasionally, when I have the privacy, but I've never been able to have an orgasm. I have had intercourse with only two guys. One is my brother who is seventeen years old. The other is a friend of my brother's who is eighteen years old. But I've never been able to have an orgasm with either of them. There is a guy that I date sometimes whom I feel I could have an orgasm with if I could get him to go all the way with me! I come very close to having an orgasm when I fantasize about him. I'll call him D. In my fantasies, D. and I start out doing stuff like eating at a nice restaurant or something. Then we go to one of our houses and start drinking. We usually drink rum and coke. After about the third drink, D. starts kissing me and playing with my breasts and stuff like that. This is where the fantasy begins, because in reality, that's where we leave off. We're lying on the sofa, and I become very horny and so does he. We undress and go into a bedroom where we make love, usually with at least the bedside lamp on. I dream that I have at least three orgasms and that we make love again the next morning.

Then I have a fantasy in which a total stranger comes to my door and I seduce him. Although I have adequate breasts (36C), in my fantasies I usually have very large, round breasts. My hair is usually very long and has lots of body.

I have one fantasy in which I am a stripteaser in a burlesque show. In my fantasy, I come out on the stage in a long red low-cut dress with a slit up the side to the base of my hip. My hair is jet black and nearly to my hips. I start doing a very seductive dance, all the men begin to whistle and applaud, and there are a few in the front row that have erections! I begin by taking off my long red gloves, next I take off my large loop earrings. Then I take off my shoes. I then open the slit to reveal the end of a garter and the top of my hose. (The garter belt is red also.) I open the slit just wide enough for the men to see that I have on NO panties. Then I close the slit, do a few more seductive moves; then I undo one strap, which really gets the men going. I undo the other strap, and then I begin to unzip the dress (it zips on the side of the slit). I very slowly unzip it. But even then I'm not nude. I have on the garter, stockings, and red strapless bra! I slowly continue to undress, teasing the men a lot! Finally, when I am nude, a man from the audience (front row) can no longer control himself. He runs up and throws me down on the stage and begins fucking me! All the other men in the audience masturbate themselves or each other. There are variations to this and all my other fantasies.

Another one that I have is one in which I'm raped! I've never fantasized about strangers or dogs though. Most of the time, the men in my fantasies are men I happen to be attracted to at that time! I find myself many times looking at the crotches of men's pants, just as I find men gazing at my breasts!

I feel that I have certain lesbian tendencies, because my first fantasies were of other girls, and sometimes I'll still have a fantasy of a girl or woman. I also find that I get excited when I see pictures of nude women! If I ever had the opportunity for a lesbian experience, I doubt that I would pass it up. But I could never be totally lesbian.

Right now, I'm looking for a nice, somewhat older man who will teach me all I need to know about sex, for I am very inexperienced and dumb. If you know anyone like this, send him my way!

I've always had sexual fantasies, and for a long time, I thought they were abnormal and weird, and I tried to suppress them. But I don't anymore.

I hope I have helped your research just a little bit. I am looking forward to your next book. Thanks again for *My Secret Garden*.

Molly

I *love* you! Having just read *My Secret Garden*, I feel compelled to write to you.

I just this moment finished the book, and I have so many jumbled thoughts that I'll try to relate my feelings to you in some orderly fashion.

First, I'm still turned on. Your book had an enormous erotic effect on me. Need I say that I had to stop numerous times to masturbate. But, oddly enough, my OWN erotic fantasies are still much more exciting to me than simply reading others.

117

I have never felt guilty about fantasizing during masturbation—I always considered that quite natural and have been doing so ever since I started masturbating regularly at age five. But I got the *greatest* relief in reading that other women regularly fantasize while fucking. I always felt terribly *guilty* about fucking one man and thinking about another. Now I realize it's not abnormal or unfair or a put-down of the guy I'm with—it just makes everything more enjoyable. What a great discovery and a great release. Thank you!

The other delightful result is that I feel closer to other women. Wouldn't it be great if we could all discuss these things with each other, rather than reading it in a book? Maybe now I will. It really allows me to feel more open to other women.

Two other minor points. I've always been an inveterate crotch-watcher, and I love it when I see some guy with a partial erection. I am delighted to find that I'm not alone. Also, sometimes I fantasize fondling and sucking another woman's breasts, and I always look at breasts. I'm glad this is also common, as I always feared I was harboring some deeply hidden lesbian tendencies. Now I know this isn't so and that my fantasy is quite common and natural.

I have only one objection. On the back of the paperback edition there is a quote from Dr. Leonard Cammer saying that fantasy "allows a needed escape from unfulfilled reality." Bullshit! He completely missed the whole point of your book—it ENHANCES reality and is NOT an escape. Typical sexist comment from a male who really does not understand women.

Thank you, Nancy, for allowing me to feel better about myself. *Everyone* should read your book.

P.S. I am college-educated, thirty, single.

Jackie

I've just finished *My Secret Garden*. Thank you very much for collecting these fantasies. Reading the book has made me feel much more at ease about the normalcy of my own fantasies.

(Incidentally, I am twenty-six years old, white, middle-class background, with three and a half years of college, and in training as a medical assistant at the moment.)

Although I am an imaginative person, I often take my fantasies whole from other sources, such as movies (not dirty movies, curiously enough, because I find them unimaginative and tasteless), novels (*The Story of O*, etc.), and other popular media.

But much more commonly, I make them up from experiences that I have had, embellished and elaborated to fantasy proportions. One of my favorites, incidentally, is about prostitution, an empty room in *My Secret Garden*.

Some years ago, I met a man who, I discovered shortly, was a bounding cad, but he was so egotistical, with *very* little reason for being so, incidentally, that I was fascinated by his conceit and was intimate with him for some months before my fascination turned to boredom at his boorish predictability, and I subsequently dropped him.

My prostitution fantasy about this man, whom I'll call Roger, goes more or less like this: I'm in the city on some important errand when I see Roger and, worse, he sees me. From his smile as he approaches, I know he means no good. Rather then create a scene, I allow him to take me into a sleazy-looking café. There he tells me he has discovered some awful thing about me, something that could ruin my personal and professional life, as well as those of my family. I think, in my fantasy, that he wants to blackmail me for money, but discover instead he intends to prostitute me for his own profit. I am helpless and must obey.

He has apparently had all this planned out, because when I follow him to his apartment, he gives me a see-through blouse, microminiskirt, black net stockings, and a black garter belt to exchange for my street clothes. But before I do this, he makes me shave my entire body, including pubic hair.

When I'm ready and dressed, we walk through downtown on our way to a party, where he has sold my services. We stop before a store with a facade that reads Novelties, but I can see by the equipment in the window that it's really a sex shop, one that sells pornographic books, and has the trappings of fetish-oriented sex. We go inside. Behind the counter is a handsome young Oriental (in real life several of my lovers have been Orientals, and I admit a preference for them over Caucasian men). He smiles at us and can tell at once by my costume and makeup what I am.

Roger ignores me and begins talking to the storekeeper about various of his goods, while I wander about and look at all the stuff hanging on the walls, such as leather harnesses, dildos, chains, whips, vibrators, etc., which makes me very hot and excited, as well as a big selection of dirty books. (This excitement, incidentally, is very odd, because I've tried some of the equipment mentioned above and was totally turned off by it, but in my fantasy, I'm so excited I bite my lips to keep from caressing myself while both men watch me.) Roger sees this and calls me over. There's a bunch of equipment on the counter that Roger wants to buy, but he doesn't have enough money. He suggests to the storekeeper that he can use me as he likes in exchange for the equipment. The storekeeper smiles again and pulls the shades to the store windows.

Roger lifts my skirt and opens my blouse, playing with me and showing me off to the storekeeper, who suggests we go upstairs. In a room upstairs, we find an enormous Newfoundland dog, and both men lay me back on the table and let the dog lick my naked mound, burrowing his big nose in as deep as he can. While the dog is doing this, Roger begins to dildo me anally. The mixture of pleasure and pain is so great I cry out noisily, which excites Roger even more and makes him go at it even more fiercely.

Quite suddenly, the Oriental pushes both the dog and Roger away from me and, taking his clothes off quickly, begins to make love to me. Roger becomes very angry and would interfere, but the storekeeper speaks in Chinese to the dog, who turns to Roger and keeps him at bay. Roger becomes furious as he helplessly watches me responding to the shopkeeper with my whole being, and not grudgingly as I did to him. I take great joy in fellating this gentle man and let him have anal intercourse, which in this case doesn't hurt as it usually does. I am aching with desire by the time he switches to plain, straight intercourse. During all this, my lover turns to Roger and says that if he (Roger) bothers or threatens me anymore, he'll suffer for it. Roger, coward that he is, believes it and slinks from the room with the growling dog at his heels. And it is this man's lovemaking and not Roger's cold-hearted fucking that swiftly brings me to one intolerably delicious orgasm on the heels of another.

And there's the basic form of one of my favorite fantasies, with true lust triumphant and the villain foiled again.

Again, with gratitude and wishes of success.

☐ I believe sex is all pervasive in the human mind and body. While we are buying groceries, we notice how handsome the clerk in the supermarket may be; women write to me of sexual fantasies they have had about their dentist while he was drilling their teeth. But we need a focus, a concrete symbol, picture, or book to make us aware and comfortable about our free-flowing sexuality. "Since I read your book, and also while reading it," writes Sally, "I began to think about my own fantasies. I always had these thoughts, since I was around twelve, but never told anyone. . . ."

Marylou tells us that she herself denied ever having sexual fantasies until she read *Garden*. "No," she told her friends when the subject came up; she never had fantasies. "I just think about my lover." But little flashbacks were registering in her head, she says, even while she denied that erotic images danced in her imagination. "When I read [*My Secret Garden*], it dawned on me just like it did on Paula in the book—oh, 'a fantasy is something that makes you feel good.' In fact, most every scene in the book has run through my fantasies but with a different script."

Marylou is an illustration of the fact that we all know more than we consciously want to know. A great deal of sexual imagery, daydreaming, reveries, and fantasy are suspended somewhere in the back of our mind. It is all like some data bank, where specific bits of information can be quickly brought forward into consciousness when the right lever is pushed, and then so quickly wheeled back after use that it is difficult to remember the thought was ever there to begin with. In this way, we live with our mental fires banked, our sexuality turned down low. Perhaps this is necessary to get through the ordinary business of the ordinary day, a necessary sacrifice of our erotic selves on the altar of an industrial society. Still—aren't these days half-unlived? I believe any stimulation is a positive good; anything that makes us feel more alive is an absolute benefit. If an occasional glance at a photo in a magazine, an image on the television screen or a page in a book makes us feel more intensely, isn't that life itself? □

Sally

At a suggestion from my sister, I have just finished reading your book. I truly thought it was fantastic. I just couldn't put it down.

First, let me tell you about myself. I am nineteen, just married last December, and I love sex. My husband is twenty-four and very healthy.

Since I read your book, and also while I was reading it, I began to think about my own fantasies. I always had these thoughts, since I was around twelve, but never told anyone or acted them out. I guess I never really thought about them until I read that other women had the same sort of thoughts.

My husband says the kind of sex we have now is fine for him, and he won't discuss his fantasies. I would like to discuss mine and several of the others I read about in your book—just talk about them, that's all—but he doesn't seem to get into it.

I don't masturbate, but often think about it. Perhaps if I read a really good book on masturbation, or someone discussed it openly with me, I would try it. When I think of another woman fingering me and eating me, it excites me intensely. It has never happened, but it sure sounds good. I also think about big masculine men, like the kind you see in *Playgirl* and *Viva*; I like to think of them stepping right out of the pages, forcefully tearing my clothes off and tying me, spread-eagle, arms apart, to the bedposts. As I look at those photos, I imagine him teasing me, fingering me to get me going, and then teasing me with just the head of his cock. I don't know where I get these ideas, as these are not things my husband does to me—I mean, teasing me with his cock. I am sure I have read about it somewhere. In my fantasy, this man from the pages of *Playgirl* then lick. my tits and belly button until I plead with him to fuck me, and at last he does. I don't think of these things when my husband and I are making love, or doing sixty-nine, but when I am alone reading porno books. Then it really turns me on. I can really throw myself into the pages of a good book. It sets my imagination going and allows me to imagine myself involved in a sexual world I am sure I will never know. All the men and women in my fantasies are faceless. They are always strangers. And even I am not recognizable; the things I allow myself to do are so unlike me. But how I would love to enjoy the thrills of the things I have read and seen on the printed page!

It's great to read how other women think, and it's stupid of me to think we aren't entitled to all the sexual excitement we can feel in our imaginations. The men that think we aren't capable of this kind of excitement must know some pretty dumb chicks.

Thanks so much.

Marylou

I just finished your book, and I wanted to tell you that I enjoyed it, and it helped me out.

My girl friend brought the book to me at a picnic. The women who were there—average midtwenties, early thirties, public schoolteachers like myself—denied having fantasies. I denied it too—"No, I just think about my lover—I've never had fantasies," but little flashbacks were registering in my head that I just couldn't put my finger on. When I read *My Secret Garden*, it dawned on me just like it did on Paula in the book—oh, "a fantasy is something that makes you feel good." In fact, most every scene in the book has run through my fantasies but with a different script. It amused me to even read in the Quickie section that two different women get their kicks from Tarzan. He was my earliest fantasy man. Everytime I read Tarzan comics, I'd get a tingle; then I'd make up my own stories before I fell asleep at night. I guess I was about twelve. I later changed to some fantasy boys—Spin and Marty. I suppose because I could then be included in the story. I daydreamed a lot at school too, but I can't remember if they were sexual types of things. I would imagine, because this pattern continued—nighttime stories and daydreaming—until I got married. I remember riding the bus to work, in my early twenties, fantasizing. My scripts were not very spicy, I don't believe. They were repressed, and I was sexually frustrated. I had engaged in every form of foreplay with boyfriends since I was fifteen, but didn't actually have intercourse till I was twenty-three. It all made me feel guilty, but the fantasies didn't.

I thought my fantasies stopped when I got married

124

seven years ago, until I read your book. But I have them more than ever. For almost three years, I've had a real lover, and he is my fantasy husband. When I go to parties at his house, I always feel and act as the hostess. And when I go home with my real husband, I go to bed with my fantasy husband. When he dances with his wife at these parties, we look at each other in the mirror over the bar, and we are really in each other's arms. He is a great fantasizer himself. On our once-a-week sessions in bed together, my lover and I sometimes fantasize together. Sometimes our motel room has two double beds in it, and we talk about the other couple making love in the other bed. Sometimes we pretend we're making a porno film. I really don't know why I said I don't have sexual fantasies.

When I masturbate, I sometimes dress in sexy clothes and watch myself in the mirror. Sometimes I use different garden vegetables. I go outside and pick a nicely proportioned zuccini squash.

I'm going to make more use of my fantasies now, instead of repressing them. It seems to me that without fantasies sex is mechanical and less fun. My husband and I rarely make love since I've started my affair. I don't want to leave him. We have a lot in common, but we can't talk like my lover and I do. I think it's unrealistic to expect one man to be Mr. Right. It takes many people to fulfill one person's needs. That sounds so exploitive. I like to think of myself as fulfilling my own needs, but I need love, someone to understand, and I need money so I can have my beautiful house in the country and my stable of horses. I'd have to live in an apartment on my teaching salary.

Best wishes on writing your new book. I'm sorry I couldn't write specific details of fantasies. They are too repressed at this point, and besides I am an artist. Words have never been my thing.

My lover should be calling soon. We have a great adventure ahead with my new viewpoint on fantasies.

CHAPTER FOUR

FRUSTRATION

☐ When I began writing *My Secret Garden*, I said, "Let's get frustration out of the way first." It is one of the great misconceptions many people have that sexual fantasies are the lonely dreamings of withered-prune old maids. This is just not true.

While the women in this section are here because in one form or another they all feel frustration in their lives, only Laura can be called a virgin—but from her description of her activities, it is clear that she remains one only technically, only by centimeters. Biba too comes close to the conventional idea of frustration. She is very close to term in her third pregnancy and writes that when fucking becomes uncomfortable, she uses masturbation and fantasy to take its place.

More often, however, it is my feeling that it is not so much the lack of sex that leads to the frustration of the women who write me as it is that the quality of their sexual experience is not all it might be. Until recently, this unhappiness was unspoken. In our culture, it was silently agreed that any woman lucky enough to have a man had no right to complain.

Contrary to popular belief, I think that as women gain more sexual freedom, we will find greater sexual frustration. Until recently, young women were so preoccupied with hanging onto their virginity that their consequent frustration was practically a badge of virtue. If you turned and tossed in your little single bed at night, at least you had the dream of keeping that symbolic rosebud that mother assured you would make you all the more cherished "when the right man comes along."

Frustration was something a "good girl" suffered silently with a Doris Day smile. Nice women just didn't talk about or, until recently, didn't even admit to themselves the genuine emotional loneliness and physical pain that can be felt by a woman who is ready and eager for sex, but is deprived of it. (Even before she has had it, she already knows she misses it. Her fantasies have told her so.)

The pill hasn't changed "everything." Throughout this book, you will find letters from women in their twenties who tell me they are still virgins. So were their mothers. But what *is* different today is that an enormous amount of information on the pleasures of sex is not only available to women but is practically inescapable: films and television do not let us forget that others are in sexual ecstasy.

Another little-discussed aspect of liberation that leads to the sexual frustration of many young women is, ironically enough, our greater freedom of selection. The most enterprising of the new generation of women no longer feel pushed or rushed into marriage. Perhaps they want a career; perhaps they simply don't want to settle for the first man who comes along. Women value themselves more, and as we do so, we are becoming more selective about men. A job you like, work you find satisfying—something to do that you feel is important—is, I believe, essential to a good life. Not only is it fulfilling in its own right but it also helps you resist the demands of our culture to marry just because you're approaching twenty-five or thirty.

But becoming your own woman, becoming highly educated and choosy in your sexual tastes, leaves you vulnerable to loneliness. You can be a virgin and be sexually frustrated. But every experienced woman knows that to have had sex, good sex, and then to have to do without it, leaves even more room for real pain.

In our culture, the pain a woman suffers from sexual deprivation isn't considered seriously. Not so with men.

The myth says, "Men are different." Men *must* have sex. His wife is frigid, or away in the country—almost any excuse suffices to "drive" a man to this or that sexual peccadillo. Society condones a frustrated man getting sex any way he can. Prostitution was created for him.

But a woman? The idea of a woman being driven to adultery, homosexuality, male prostitution (if she can find it)=these notions make us shudder. It is thought demeaning of a woman to express such strong sexual desires. "She needs it bad" is not a sexual compliment; it is a put-down. And yet why should it be thought that women suffer any less than men from going without sex? We may not wake up in the morning with an erection or out of a wet dream, but we dream, and we fantasize out of lack of sex. We suffer as much from it as any man.

As for married women and sexual frustration, I think we are just beginning to comprehend the toll that sexless, or sexually unimaginative, marriages have taken on women. Women like Lyle are just beginning to cry out against the unfairness or sexual immaturity of a husband who prefers masturbation to her. She is contemporary enough to say she doesn't have anything against him jerking off, except in the way that it cheats her. But her acceptance of her husband's habits does her no good. She is left with very imaginative, but lonely, fantasies. □

Laura

First I ought to explain that I'm a seventeen-year-old virgin. I masturbate almost every day, frequently go out petting with guys, and love to suck guys off.

Some of my sexual fantasies are of specific things that have happened. I lay there and try to recreate in my imagination some of the sensations I have felt. I love to think of slipping my hand down a guy's unzipped

128

pants and feeling his hair, reaching the obstacle of the top of his cock, and feeling his cock grow. I remember the feeling of his skin sliding as I move my hand up and down. I like the familiar feeling of a guy rolling over on top of me (both of us nude), his erect cock pressed against my stomach—it's probably the temptation (so near, yet so far) that makes it so exciting. I remember individual gestures, bedroom jokes, and the smells I enjoyed—wine or pot on his breath, slight sweatiness, and after-shaves. Each of these thoughts is a small glimpse rather than a total experience.

My masturbatory fantasies are pieced together out of these thoughts, and assigned to some particular person. One of my fantasies is of sucking off Bjorn Borg, the Swedish tennis player. I think of the slippery rubberiness of his cock, the soft wetness of the tip, the feel of the pulsations at the base of his cock as he comes, and the taste of semen. After I developed this fantasy, I read in *Playgirl* that most Scandinavians are uncircumsised. That made the fantasy even more exciting.

It excites me to see a guy get a hard-on in public. I start fantasizing about sex with him, even if I would never previously have considered it.

Two guys once wanted to have sex with me. I turned them down, and took them one at a time. Now I think about group sex, but I wouldn't consider it if another girl was there.

I have a fetish about guys who have weird hair. Kinky, wavy, or curly hair is a big turn-on.

I also fantasize about screwing, with details being guessed—I just assume that most of the feelings are nearly identical to those of being petted, except the penis is larger and harder to control (putting pressure in certain areas, the degree of pressure, speed, etc.).

I keep fantasizing, but since most of my sex is with guys that I don't know well (I like them, but I don't want their kids or their v.d.), I'm not ready yet to take responsibility for screwing.

I'm looking for a guy who enjoys pleasing me as much as I enjoy pleasing him (and if Bjorn wants my address . . .).

Thanks for letting me express myself. I didn't think I was abnormal for having fantasies, only that I was abnormal for admitting it.

P.S. If there's nothing far out about my fantasies, maybe I represent the young and inexperienced.

Biba

You have no mention of pregnant women in your book of fantasies.

My third baby is due in two weeks. I am masturbating and fantasizing a lot. It started in the fourth month. I think it is because actual fucking is uncomfortable about then and became more so as I progressed.

During my first and second pregnancy my masturbating and fantasizing increased too. I was married to someone else then. He was big and hurt me. I gave up normal sex willingly in the last six weeks. I would jerk him off though. I liked his bigness when I wasn't pregnant. He couldn't satisfy me emotionally though.

My husband now I love dearly. He is not so big and more flexible, so I am still willing to have sex, even now. He holds off as long as he can, because the baby does react violently. Also, because of the positions we have to take. He enters from behind, or I will throw one leg over his hips while he is on his side; I on my back. This does not allow much penetration, so he has to be really horny to climax. I can't climax no matter how horny he makes me feel or how much I wish I could. So I will tell how I get relieved. I am always alone and my children asleep.

I start out playing with my nipples, in front of the mirror. My hands become some girl's hand, pinching, tweaking, kneading, cupping. Soon it is two girls, one for each breast. My breasts are really big now, so I can actually get a nipple in my mouth and suck, imagining the girls are the ones sucking me. A third girl comes in from behind, she grabs my ass, massaging around and around. She kisses my butt and puts her tongue to my anus, slurping. A fourth girl kneels down in front of me and starts kissing the inside of my legs, up, up, coming ever closer to my vagina. I spread my legs even further apart for her. She slowly sucks my cunt, moving just right on my lips, my clitoris. A fifth girl appears sitting on the vanity. Her legs spread apart. I move to suck her tits. The girl between my legs is sucking oh so good. I go down on the girl sitting in front of me, sucking her cunt. The girls sucking my tits reach their hands to caress the tits of the girl I'm sucking, also to the tits of the girl at my ass. I reach out my arms and finger their pussies. The girl between my legs is about to make me climax. I then move to the bed, put a pillow between my legs, and masturbate to a climax within seconds, still imagining I have a girl between my legs, at my ass, sucking my tits, around my fingers, and in my mouth.

Sometimes I look at pictures of nude girls to start this fantasy, and look at her when I get to masturbating.

I have never had a girl eat me out or have I eaten someone. This type of fantasy entered my mind during my first pregnancy.

Men have eaten me out; some were really good.

I would like to be able to have normal sex real bad. I can hardly wait until the time I can climax right along with my husband.

Lyle

Nancy Friday, you are some kind of genius! Thank you for putting together such an inspirational, interesting book.

I am twenty-five, of Scandinavian and American Indian

stock, and have a large frame but not fat. I was married three years ago, and am considering *not* staying married to him for a number of reasons, the LEAST of which is this—he is a lousy lay. He is thirty-two.

On the surface, I think he is a nice man, but to live with him is very frustrating and seems an eighty-twenty balance instead of fifty-fifty—or at least a bearable sixty-forty. What I mean is I do too much of the giving, and no matter how I try to get him to "give" in this relationship, he just won't put up with the realities of loving, sharing, talking, making plans, and all the other things two married people are SUPPOSED to share as a couple.

My man was introduced to sex in a whorehouse in Nevada, and from now until then, he has had quite a few women and hasn't learned a darned thing. Before we were married, he used to tell me how horny he was. What a laugh. He might feel horny, but he's horny for his own hand. I guess no woman's pussy has ever been able to take the place of his own technique.

The first time I discovered he was masturbating on a more or less regular basis was the first year we were married. His aroused moments waned, and I just chalked it up to studying too hard . . . it never entered (and still doesn't) my mind that there was anything wrong with me. I keep myself clean and fresh, attractive in a wholesome way, and have never turned him away when he wanted me. Anyway, I was sorting laundry and noticed some funny-looking hankies of his. The ironed creases were still in them, but they were stuck together in the middle. He had come into them. I was so shocked and hurt; it was like a slap in the face, like saying I wasn't good enough to make love to, but I was sure good enough to clean up after him! Had he been in our place when I found those, I would have crammed them (still makes me mad) down his throat. In further inspection of the laundry, I found two undershirts and some more hankies which pretty well explained his lack of desire for me—the fool had worn himself out. I could have thrown up. He was a student at this time. I work, he worked part-time.

I confronted him with this little passion of his and told him how hurt I was. He said he wouldn't do it anymore, but that was a lie—evidence to the contrary shows he is still a careless man only in love with his hand.

His lovemaking with me is stilted, inhibited, and very boring. He never wants to try a different position, and I practically have to beg him to let me go down on him. I have never forced him to do anything, but have made some suggestions, all of them met with no enthusiasm whatsoever. He has never touched my vagina more than two minutes and doesn't bother to search and caress my clitoris. By the way, when he does let me fellate him, he won't come until he pushes me away, throws me down, and then gets on top of me. Jesus, I'm dying for some variation!

I have tried to deal with this patiently, never begged him to do kinky things, and never forced myself on him. He is really repulsed by women's advances. Older women who are making tries at flirting with younger men really turn him off. Instead of taking it as a compliment and giving the ladies a wink (that's all I'd ever approve of!) he just gets hostile.

With this short summary of how I feel about him, I think you will see that I have reasons a-plenty for my fantasies.

After reading your first book about these fantasies, I searched my mind for when I first awakened to that wondrous warm feeling in my pelvis, and I think it happened when I was playing doctor and nurse with my brother and one of his friends. I was totally fascinated with the wrinkled scrotum that held their testicles. I still love to gently caress that precious place with my tongue.

A few of my girlhood friends and I just loved to tell each other what excited us and sometimes touch each other "where it felt good." We could really think up some whoppers of fantasies, but we had never seen ANY-THING in our fantasies such as the large penises which so frequently dominated the stóries. We passed right on into dating without any qualms about our little experiences. I guess we just figured it was "practice" for the real thing. I never even thought about it in a lesbian connotation after I found out what lesbians were.

Since I still find my husband's careless "reminders" that Portnoy, masturbator champion of the world, lives here, I have really let the fantasies help me out when he does (rare occasions) want me.

A few years ago (before marriage), I had an affair with a man who worked in my building. He was fantastic in bed. I just wished we had been able to let ourselves get into a better relationship, such as married! Anyway, this dark-haired man would excite me into dynamite climaxes. I didn't know the human body could stand such pleasure. I swear, the first time he ate me I thought I had died and gone to heaven! I long for someone to do it again, so I imagine when my husband is puffing away that actually I am not suffocating under his lunging; instead, a large-framed man with full lips and big black eyes like my former lover is caressing my thighs and telling me how much he loves my pale, creamy skin (which I work hard at in reality to keep that way). He caresses closer to my pussy, gives me a loving, tender, but devilish gaze, and with a rich mellow laugh of glee proceeds tenderly to bring me to the heavenly feeling of pure climax. I just love putting this down on paper.

As he goes on, I have a couple of wonderful orgasms; he turns me around and straddles my face, so we can be sixty-nine together, and I can bring him joy also. That fantasy is about the greatest one for me, but sometimes I vary and use these.

I am caressing myself alone one evening as the sun sets. A girl friend of mine is due, and when she arrives, I let her in, and she sees I am naked. Immediately, she knows what I want, and she says she wants me too, so we proceed to my large (fantasy) canopy bed and slip between silk sheets edged with yards and yards of ruffles. We cover every inch of each other's bodies with kisses and do cunnilingus on each other, arriving at marvelous orgasms together.

I imagine I am alone in the high mountain cottage of the Alps, or someplace where the air is perfectly pure, standing on my balcony in a dress of white. My breasts are exposed, and the crisp air makes my nipples stand out hard and makes me feel alive to breathe it in so deeply.

A very handsome, healthy man walks by and sees me on my balcony. He says he is overwhelmed by the look of me, and asks without embarrassment if he may come up to my room and admire me closer. I gaze down on him, see the bulge growing in his pants, and with a toss of my thick head of hair say, "Of course, I'll make us some tea," and give him the warmest smile I can manage. He enters my room, which is mirrored on one wall and papered in purple and blue Jacobean floral design on the others. Many pillows are used in the room, and purple, blue, pink, and red are the dominant colors. He opens my white dress to my navel and admires my lovely skin and healthy body. Then he can stand it no longer, so he picks me up and carries me to the bed, and we make love in many different positions, all possible because he has a beautiful long penis that is surrounded by a mass of black hair, and that penis just won't give up until we are both laughing and practically hysterical with happiness and climaxes.

I don't want you to think I have anything against masturbation, like I said about my husband earlier. I think it is great, but not when it deprives someone else (like your mate) of the passion and lovemaking they need.

Thanks for letting me write this down. Hope it helps some in your next edition.

P.S. Sorry for all the typos, but I'm a writer, and I

knew I would redo too much to keep the freshness of my thoughts. So here it is . . . in the rough.

☐ If you think the kind of marital despair that Lyle suffers is rare, speak to any experienced marriage counselor. In our culture, a woman is supposed to be complete when she has a husband, a nice house, kids, station wagon, and so forth. How dare she cry for more? If her husband is working himself to death (his own, but also the death of sex between them)—it only shows what a good husband and father he is. The fact that she may have unappeased sexual desires of her own—and her a mother!—is unacceptable.

"A lot of men are coming in completely bewildered by all the new demands being made on them," says Dr. Salvatore Ambrosino, director of the Family Service Association serving Nassau County, a plush suburb outside New York City. "Women are getting a whole new picture of themselves," he said. "Through feminism and maybe even consciousness-raising sessions, they are getting the idea that they are allowing themselves to be willing victims, and they are protesting."

Dr. Ambrosino continues: "Women used to put up with a lot as long as the man was a good provider, but no more. This applies even to working-class women. We rarely used to hear complaints about women not being sexually satisfied . . . now we do." (*New York Times,* October 16, 1974.)

The final, tough fact we must face is that even with the sexiest lover or husband in the world, a woman may still find herself frustrated. Dot tells us that she has had a very active and satisfying sex life for ten years with a wide variety of lovers, but her fantasies are all about sex with another woman. To some degree, most of us, women and men, suffer some sense of frustration. Buried deep, or not-so-deep, within us all, there are tastes, desires, strange longings, and erotic images left over from the polymorphous perverse period of infancy and childhood; these constantly seek and find expression in various kinds of rich and varied foreplay, or in fantasies like Dot's.

In our adult years, frustration comes in many forms. We may choose to let certain sexual opportunities pass, because we essentially believe in monogamy . . . because the proposition was made in an unappealing manner or in terms we found emotionally sterile . . . maybe simply because we did not have the time. But each opportunity is registered in your brain and unconscious somewhere. Very often, we find fantasies are born out of the very experiences we found the most degrading or repellent in our everyday lives.

Even if you quit your job, obtained a divorce, had a million dollars in the bank, and devoted the rest of your life to erotic pursuits (a common fantasy), it would still be impossible for anyone to handle all the sexual stimuli that surround us every day. Who could make love to every attractive man she meets? When you choose one, you are letting all the rest go by. Even if you tried, there is still the persistent knowledge that while you may be systematically trying out the best lovers for fifty miles around, there are still handsome, beautiful men walking the streets of London, Paris, Rome—marvelous men, astonishing lovers who you will never meet, never know. Desire is long; life is short. We live with a residue of unspent desire—"something gone, something missed, a door closed forever."

It is not the mere quantity of sex that can still the ache in our heart. We long for a quality of sex we have never known, will never know in this life. In a world that has lost religion, *orgasm* is perhaps the last mystic experience we can believe in. We look to it for a kind of transcendence we no longer can find in church on Sunday. It is too heavy a load of expectation for even sex to bear.

Frustration is the result. Many of our fantasies are the result of using our imagination to make up for experiences we may never have. Rather than saying that these fantasies grow out of sexual impoverishment, I would say they express a desire for greater sexual richness, and are themselves a form of erotic munificence. They do not express the lack of sex, but are sex in themselves.

Gloria writes that "my new lover is my sexual *ideal,* shows me positions I've never heard of. Nor is he inhibited about talking during or after sex, and asks me about what turns me on, or how something feels." He is so secure in his masculinity, she says, that "Maybe one day I'll tell him about my fantasies. . . . He feels no need to prove anything to anyone, which is one of the reasons I love him more than anyone."

I submit the proposition that Gloria is far from a conventionally frustrated woman; but even in the midst of this sexual paradise in which she lives, she still wants something more. Although she is in love with this "ideal" man, she *can* imagine somebody else: a younger man. What I find particularly interesting in Gloria's letter is that it shows she would also enjoy a switch in roles. Her sexually knowing lover is always teaching her new positions and ideas—which she loves; with her seventeen-year-old virgin fantasy lover, *she* is the one who is the initiator, the skilled, expert partner who introduces the boy into pleasures he never had before. □

Dot

I just finished reading *My Secret Garden.* I think it is one of the best books on this topic. It is written very plain and simple, without a lot of confusion.

I fantasize twenty-four hours a day (awake and sleeping), and have since I was twelve years old (I am now twenty-eight). I was starting to think I was abnormal until I read your book. I am single and have had a very active sex life for about the last ten years with various lovers, all married. The only thing I think about when I am making love is how wonderful it feels; there is nothing that can compare to it. I do masturbate almost every day, sometimes a couple of times a day. I love to do this when reading a sexy book or looking at pictures of naked women. So I guess most of my fantasies are lesbian, although I have never had an affair with another woman. I like to lay in bed at night and think what it would be like to have a woman make love to me. I love to feel my nipples get hard and think about how it would feel to have a woman suck on them. I play with myself until I reach a orgasm, and at the same time imagine someone is eating me. I also like to think about doing the same things to someone else. As much as I love doing this and thinking about it and maybe someday having an affair with a woman, I never would want to replace a man. That is the best fucking there is. I also think about what it would be like to have both a man and a woman making love to me at the same time. I have never told anyone about my fantasies before, and I feel relieved that I can write it to someone (also very horny right now).

Thank you again for a great book.

Gloria

I feel as if I can address you by your first name, since you shared with me and your other readers such an intimate part of yourself. Right now I am lying on a bed, with your book in front of me. For some reason, none of my fantasies, except for one shortly alluded to, is in your book.

I am one of those people who do not fantasize while making love; I more or less lose consciousness instead, being aware only of physical sensations. I do fantasize when I am bored, or horny and alone. Although I consider myself *very* sophisticated sexually (nothing ever surprised me), I'm just finding out some new things now. My new lover is my sexual *ideal*, shows me positions I've never heard of. Nor is he inhibited about talking during or after sex, and asks me about what turns me on, or how something feels. Maybe one day I'll tell him about my fantasies, since he's one of the few men who are really secure about their masculinity. He feels no need to prove anything to anyone, which is one of the reasons I love him more than anyone.

But about my fantasies themselves. My favorite one is also the longest and most detailed.

I imagine myself driving a convertible sports car. (Speed is a sexual turn-on, something racing drivers don't admit to as a reason for liking fast driving.) Anyway, I am going about ninety miles an hour down a freeway, and I pull up beside another sports car wiith its top down, as mine is. Driving the car is an attractive boy of about seventeen. He looks over at me, grins, and speeds up his car, so that he is going as fast as I am. This willingness to play along with me and his appearance turn me on. (It only takes five minutes to arouse me to orgasm.) He turns off the same exit I do, so I begin to follow him. He is very aware of me and drives to a secluded area and pulls over to the side of the road. I pull up behind him and get out of the car immediately. I am wearing hot pants and a halter top (great legs and shoulders). I decide to handle the situation as directly as possible. When I reach his car window, I bend down close to him and say, "Driving like that is really a turn-on." He smiles at me rather shyly and agrees. Before long, we are discussing cars enthusiastically, and one topic leads to another. Soon I am sitting in his car with him, and we move closer and closer together, until we are embracing and kissing instead of talking. We become aroused quickly, and he tells me, reluctantly, that he is a virgin. I tell him that we all have to start somewhere, then invite him to come home with me; he agrees eagerly.

The next two hours are so unique to me, for I have never made love to a virgin before. I enjoy the look on his face as he enters me for the first time, and thrill to the sound of his moan and gasp when he comes. Altogether, we make love three times, and I come at least eight times. Finally, he says he must go home. He writes down my phone number before he leaves, and I know I will hear from him again.

I once came close to acting out this fantasy. I met the man the way I met the boy in my fantasy, but he was by no means a virgin, but a rather lazy, selfish lover.

I have another fantasy involving a pool under a gentle waterfall, and one in which I make love with another woman. It would not be traumatic for me to enact my fantasies in real life, as I do not fantasize about rape or sadism or anything that I wouldn't like to try sometime. I guess I don't feel even subconsciously guilty or hostile, at least not where my sexuality is concerned. I do sometimes fantasize clobbering somebody over the head with a baseball bat, but only when I'm mad at them.

I am going to read your book again, and I am looking forward to reading your second one. It would be interesting to see my fantasy printed in a book like yours, as I encourage people to become more open about this aspect of their sexuality. Perhaps, when, or if, men are able to accept this aspect of women, we will be able to better understand each other on all levels.

I was impressed by your openness and philosophy of liking yourself. I believe self-acceptance is one of the true keys to happiness with one's life, which is why I am not ashamed to give my real name. Thanks and best wishes for success with your next book.

Please excuse the odd handwriting, but I am stoned, which allowed me to be honest.

☐ One of the great needs that sexual fantasy fulfills for a woman is that of foreplay. Fantasy helps us reach that level of arousal he is at already . . . or he wouldn't have invited us into the bedroom to begin with. In a more egalitarian society, it will not matter if the man or the woman is the sexual initiator; if one is in the mood and the other is not, there will be no great feeling of rejection, because the roles can as easily be switched next time.

Right now, however, given the male-oriented rules under which we live, it is usually the man who gets the action going *when he's ready*. Almost conspiratorially, women go along with this idea, perpetuating the myth of man as the lusty beast who must half-coax, half-wrestle his powerless, shy maiden into bed. In her heart, every woman knows how incomplete this picture is.

It doesn't take into account the times when she's lusty as hell, and he's a hundred miles away, or times when he's panting like a bull, and she has a roast in the oven, the children to pick up in an hour, or simply her mind on other things. But the cold hand that grips the heart of America when we see a wife in some television drama unwittingly reject a sexually aroused husband grips our own hearts when our husband/lover reaches for us and we start to push him away. "You just don't do that to a man!" is the sampler mother silently stitched in our brains. The "correct" thing is to let the roast burn, your own work go undone, and, yes, fake pleasure and orgasm if you don't feel like it. Satisfy his lust if you love him, because there is something mysteriously unexplained about what will happen to the male ego if he is sexually rejected. It's not just that he'll get warts on his scrotum, turn to some other (probably socially diseased) woman for an outlet; what is equally awful is that we ourselves will feel less of a woman for having rejected him. Our womanliness rests on his desiring us. Our "selfishness" (as we have been trained to call it) may risk our entire future sexual happiness together. He may not try the next time; he may lose interest; something terrible and bad may happen not just to his cock as well as temporarily to his male ego but perhaps permanently to our shaky status as "real women."

To be fair, it is a lovely feeling to be surprised in the middle of a household chore, or while at the typewriter, to find that your lover has this giant erection and is dying for you. He's frantically working that damn jammed zipper, leading you toward the bedroom while covering you with kisses and fondling your breasts . . . you are pleased, laughing with pleasure and amusement and need no great urging at all. You're both enjoying his spontaneous moment together, *but you are running on different timetables.* Specifically, he's already had (or is having) his fantasy of fucking you, and is fully aroused. You are miles behind, because somewhere at the back of your mind, you're still in the middle of that complicated recipe you were following in the kitchen or unraveling that snarled paragraph in the typewriter.

The problem is further complicated by the medically documented fact that physiologically men usually reach climax sooner than women. So not only is he mentally ready for sex long before he's made you aware of his intentions but his glands and nerve endings are physically geared to race ahead of yours too. The result is that many of the most loving women often finish their sexual experiences feeling a little rushed, unsatisfied, even left out. Callie is lucky enough to have a husband who is aware of these problems. He uses sexual fantasies as a form of foreplay to ensure that his wife always reaches orgasm. In fact, he is the one who tells them to her. "The only problem," she writes about his practice of using sexual fantasies as a form of foreplay, "is that usually your mind is racing ahead of the logical progression of the story . . . many times, my husband or I are unable to reach the 'good part' . . . because the anticipation of what's to come is all that is required" . . . to reach orgasm.

Unfortunately, not many women have husbands who are prepared to go to these lengths to stimulate their wives before penetration. Arlene writes unhappily that her husband "doesn't believe in any type of foreplay at all. . . . Sex lasts a total of three minutes if we are lucky."

The thing to remember is that you have a form of foreplay available to you at a moment's notice. You carry it in your mind. Try to remember one of your favorite sexual fantasies—one that you may have read in this book, or a new one you may have invented yourself. It is a marvelous way to quickly rev yourself up to his level of excitement . . . to join or even beat him in the headlong rush to climax.

One of the ironies of fantasy is that the hero of our erotic reveries is rarely the man we love. Perhaps it is the very fulfillment and satisfaction we get from him that leaves nothing to the imagination, and so we need these strangers in the night to people our imaginary sexual worlds. They bring us the excitement of the unknown.

Arlene is one of the rare exceptions to the rule. Perhaps it is because her husband *does* leave her so unsatisfied that she says it is he who is making love to her when she masturbates. "I imagine us both climaxing together, and I almost go out of my mind with pleasure."

Her fantasies show us that Arlene is hardly a sexually insatiable or strange woman. All she is asking for is something any woman is entitled to; in one of the fantasies she has sent in, perhaps she herself has found a way to get what she wants in reality. When she masturbates, Arlene writes that she uses her hairbrush, sausages, a cucumber . . . "I think I would die if he caught me, but I sometimes imagine him walking in, and it excites me even more."

Perhaps she might be very happily surprised if she let him do just that? □

Callie

Thank you so much for *My Secret Garden.* I haven't thought that I was weird, but I have wondered if other women fantasize as much as I do. I am just forty years old and have been married for twenty-two years. Since I didn't have any relations prior to marriage and haven't had any with anyone except my husband, I have fantasized as to what it would be like.

During foreplay, my husband always masturbates me to a climax. I usually climax very easily, but at times need mental help—that's where the fantasies come in. My husband and I share them—in fact, he usually relates them to me. We have two favorites that we use at this time in our foreplay.

Fantasy 1: The brush salesman arrives. He has so many items to show, I tell him to spread them on the floor in front of the couch. I excuse myself for a moment, go to the bedroom, and remove my panties. I am wearing a miniskirt, so as I sit on the edge of the couch to better see his display, I am quite exposed. He is kneeling on the floor. As he shows me his items, I show him mine. Whenever I reach down to pick up a brush, I carelessly open my thighs. I watch his eyes out of the corner of mine, and he is practically staring at my exposed cunt. I increase the exposure. He finally takes a chance and mentions something appropriate. I act semishocked. He says he will be gentle and logically adds that I must want him to otherwise I would have been more careful. I weaken and finally give in, but I tell him that he cannot fuck me—only my husband can do that. The best I can offer is to let him play with my cunt and suck it. He eagerly accepts. I lay back, pull my skirt all the way up, spread my legs, and he starts to move toward me. I reach down and open the lips and—I usually come now, if not before.

Fantasy 2: A variation of the first. I promise a sales appointment to a salesperson at one of those lingerie parties, in return for a hostess gift for my friend. The salesperson arrives at my house, and he is a very good-looking man. I act flustered, and he assures me that he helps women try on bras and undergarments all of the time and thinks nothing of it. I go in the bedroom and put on my robe over panties and bra. He gives me a bra to try on. I slip my robe to my waist, turn my back, and try to change bras. My robe is too hard to try to hold, and with his reassurances, I figure what the heck and let it drop. I complain of the fit—rubs and pulls in the front. He says that I probably did not lay my breasts in the cups properly. He has me lean over after he has undone the bra. He reaches under and cups my breasts while explaining how it should go and feel. While cupping my tits, he has very gently rubbed the nipples, and they are erecting. The bra fits, and I decide to take it, but after removing the demonstrater, I don't put my other one back on. I am thrilled to stand there with my lovely tits completely bare, the nipples now erected like pencil erasers, and see him looking at them. He gets out the panty hose, and I try on a pair. I again complain of the fit. He says my panties are wrinkling up under the panty hose and suggests that, for the purpose of fitting them, I should remove my panties. By now I quickly agree. After putting the panty hose back on, I look in the full-length mirror. The hose is so sheer that nothing is left to the imagination. My cunt is really quite hairy and extends up toward my belly quite a ways. I see him looking at it in the mirror over my shoulder. By now, both in and out of the fantasy, I am very hot. I tell him that it is pulling in the crotch—knowing full well what he will do. He slips his hand down the front, over my bush, and places his fingers on the lips. He moves them about and asks if that feels better. I say somewhat, but it still isn't right. He sits in a chair nearby and asks me to come over, so he can see what the problem is. As I stand inches from him, he rolls the panty hose down over my hips and on down off of one leg. He asks me to put one foot on the arm of his chair, and he will see what was bothering me. As I do this, he leans forward into my spread legs, using his fingers to open the lips, and very gently lays his tongue between them—and I come, both in the fantasy and for real.

The only problem with these fantasies is that usually your mind is racing ahead of the logical progession of the story. In that event, many times, my husband or I are unable to reach the "good part" of the story, because the anticipation of what's to come is all that is required to accomplish the purpose.

One more favorite that I usually use when I masturbate. My husband is a pilot. Of course, many layovers occur with various stewardesses. Contrary to public opinion, there doesn't seem to be much hanky-panky on these layovers. We have a good sex life, so I am sure he is not fooling around with these girls; however, I do fantasize about it while masturbating. It is very sexy to imagine him doing this. (I don't tell him this, of course.)

Fantasy 3: I get on a plane and follow him to his layover point. He has been in the hotel for a couple of hours. I get a key from the room clerk and go upstairs. I know what I will find. I open the door. He is naked and sitting in a chair, with an enormous hard-on. In front of him, standing with her hips thrust forward and one foot on the arm of the chair, is a gorgeous stewardess whom I know. She is nude. She is a big girl—but not fat. She has a beautiful body. Lovely, huge, but well-formed, tits. She is very blonde except for her cunt, which is very bushy with black hair. My husband is licking her cunt as she looks at me and smiles and invites me in. On the bed is an equally stunning brunette, also nude. She invites me to remove my clothes and tells me that, "He will be ready in a few minutes." I sit in a chair. By now, they have moved to the bed. The blonde is sucking my husband's cock. She is being sucked by the brunette, and, of course, my husband is eating the brunette's cunt. I am so hot watching them that I am now playing with my cunt and rubbing my nipples until I climax. The girls also climax, but my husband does not. The blonde finally turns to me and says, "He's ready now." I go over to the bed and slowly let myself down on that wonderful prick. The girls are beside us, going down on each other. As I watch them and ride that cock—I climax.

I have rambled on far too much I fear, but as some of your other contributors have said, it's good to be able to tell someone. Detailed fantasies are still somewhat out of place at the coffee klatch.

I believe in your sincerity, but feel more comfortable signing only my first name.

Arlene

My Secret Garden was a great book. I bought it by accident, and it turned out to be the best accident I ever had.

I am married one and a half years, and I am happy now that I read *My Secret Garden*. See, my husband has an unusual problem that's driving me insane. He doesn't believe in any type of foreplay at all, except for himself. I have to do everything to him, but he won't excite me in any way. He just mounts me and slides in and out maybe four times, and he pulls out and comes. Sex lasts a total of three minutes if we are lucky. I asked numbers of times why he won't come inside of me, but never get any answer. I am told to lay still on the bed, and when I try to move along with him, he seems to have the idea only men are supposed to enjoy sex. I put up with this every day. When he goes to work I am so overjoyed. I found myself one day lying on the bathroom floor with my hairbrush, just thinking how it would be making love to my husband. It is so beautiful I have to do it almost every day now. I imagine us both climaxing together, and I almost go out of my mind with pleasure. Then I go to the store and look for other goodies to replace my hairbrush. So far I've had a hot dog, knockwurst, sausage, cucumber. I think I would die if he caught me, but I sometimes imagine him walking in, and it excites me even more.

☐ Bunny writes that her lovemaking with her husband is "always exciting and complete. . . ." Although he is crippled and unable to walk, they have a son, and, "baby," she proudly declares of her husband, "he has more energy than a young man when it comes down to fucking. We have a lot of fire and believe me, we burn it all up. The days of Zip Zam Thank You Ma'am are all over with." Bunny's husband is as avid and experimental about sex as is Bunny herself, and yet in the very heart of Bunny's full erotic life, she names a frustration: she has always had a fantasy of making love to a woman. This is an important theme that runs through letter after letter in this book, from women in every sexual walk of life.

"Who knows better than a woman how to satisfy another woman?" I think that sentence haunts the bedroom of every woman who knows the fireworks oral sex can hold for her, but whose lover is inexperienced, unskilled, or just downright reluctant about it. Even Bunny, who never implies any lack of ardor or skill to her husband in any sexual area, found it a thrilling experience. Describing what happened when, with her husband's willing consent and participation, she put her fantasy into practice, Bunny describes the feeling of having another woman go down on her: "She had a tongue that knew every spot there is to know on a woman."

Because Bunny does not call herself a lesbian, I do not consider her one. (The fact that she is married is not, of course, evidence either way.) Some lesbians are proud of the name. Other women describe homosexual fantasies to me, but add the proviso that while they enjoy thinking about it, they nevertheless consider themselves heterosexuals. Bunny herself, in her enthusiasm and gusto for sex in all its forms, never seems to give the matter any thought at all—and I think she is probably the wisest of all. □

Bunny

I have had fantasies for years, but never gave them a second thought until my husband and I began sharing them. Now fantasies are a part of our everyday life. It all began when my husband, I, and my son took a trip to Houston, Texas, in 1972, with two other couples. When we woke up the next morning, the women decided to go shopping. We walked for about six blocks, when a peep-show store caught my eyes. I always wanted to go into one of those shops, and being away from home, I felt more at ease walking into the place. So I asked the women would they go with me. One said okay, but the other one grabbed my little boy, who was two years old, and said no, I'm not going into that place (the poor woman should have gone; she might have learned something). I was really amazed at the books, dildos of all sizes, vibrators, and French ticklers that they had on display. I went around the store trying to pick out the best books, but naturally I only could look at the cover and use my own judgment, for the books were covered in transparent wrapping. So I picked out three books that I thought would be enjoyable. I could not wait to get back to the room to open them. When I did, I could not believe my eyes. Honey, those books had me and my husband wondering what in the world had we been missing. My husband and I would look at them every chance we had. I really enjoyed the lesbian shows. When we make love, I tell my husband my fantasy about making love to a woman. Our lovemaking was always exciting and complete, and the thought of me eating a woman really aroused us more. So we made plans to get someone, to see how enjoyable it would really be. One night, a friend of ours came down. She is always talking about sex. I asked her if she ever had a woman eat her; she said no, but was indeed very curious about it. I told her about the plans me and my husband had made, and to my surprise, she was very willing. She undressed faster than we did. I had been curious for months about eating a woman, so here we were, all three of us lying there naked, and I wondering would I do a good job on her. I always knew I did a hell of a blow job on my husband, but, damn, eating a woman, shit what a difference, so I got to it. First I fondled with her breast, then slowly worked my way down with my tongue to her cunt. I opened it with a gentle touch, the way my husband opens me, ease in my hot tongue, and watched her face expression change to: Goddamn it's about time you got there! I ate her till my husband could take no more, and he began eating me. After we brought her home, we got back in bed and started where we left off. Here I had eaten this chick and I enjoyed it, but there was a problem: I wanted a woman to eat me. We have this other friend who is just eighteen, but knows a lot about sex. She came down one night. My husband had company, so she came to the bedroom. I was lying there with just my robe on watching the "Untouchables" when I felt her hand going under my robe. She is the type of person who says if you want something go after it, so I gathered she wanted my pussy, and baby she was welcome to it. She had experience. I could tell by the way her hands moved to my cunt, and she parted my lips so gently. She came closer to reach my neck and kiss it softly; then she slowly lowered her head to my pearl. Goddamn that bitch knew just what she was doing. And I enjoyed every minute or it. Then my husband joined us. It was another threesome, but this time, the woman was eating me. She had a tongue that knew every spot there is to know on a woman.

I never believed that a woman could make me feel the excitement that I felt that very minute. My husband made love to me while she blew him. Then I made love to her, while my husband fucked me from behind; then he made love to her while I blew him; then we both made love to him, she blew him while I sucked his chest. Then he fucked both of us.

Now this fantasy that I love having is about my husband's old girl friend. From the minute I met her, I always liked her. After three years of knowing her, I just found out from my husband that they were lovers before he met me. It has been a year since we saw her. She is in Europe now with her husband. Ever since I had my husband tell me how he used to make love to her, I fantasize that she comes over, and we are drinking Vodka like we used to do. I ask her if she would like my husband to eat her, and how willing she is, so we all undress. My husband is always teasing people, so he begins making love to me first, knowing how excited she would get, blowing in my ears, biting my neck, licking all over my body, then slowly parting my lips and licking my cunt, then going to my pearl. But never entering into my cunt. But then I feel a tongue entering inside of me, a long hot tongue licking every corner, catching every drop of juice that's dripping down. That chick really has her shit together, a tongue still on my pearl and a hot tongue slowly taking its time going around and around into my cunt. She and my husband give me a hell of a working over until I can't take anymore, now I need a fucking, so my husband gives her the dildo to put on. She is now working with it just at the tip of my cunt, every now and then she stabs me with it. My husband is sucking my breast and playing with my pearl. Now we begin to get more excited. She begins penetrating inside of me with the dildo. I begin shouting I'm coming bitch, just keep on working inside of me. Then my husband starts making love to her. She begins kissing me and I her. While my husband is eating her, she gets between my legs and slowly starts eating my cunt, and I start sucking my husband's prick, and we all come to climax together.

Sometime me and my husband fantasize about four men holding us up and taking us into a shed, where they fuck me while my husband is tied up and can do nothing but watch. One guy is eating me while the other one shoves his big black prick into my mouth. The other two lick all over my body. After they all eat me and I suck their pricks, a woman is brought in, and she begins to eat me, then I eat her. She is then brought over to my husband. He is untied and he begins to eat her. Now a German shepherd is brought in and he begins to lick my cunt and asshole. When his red penis begins to show, they insert it into me, and we begin fucking. Now my husband and that woman are doing sixty-nine. We all have reached our climax now, and everyone is beat as hell.

My husband and I have been married for three years.

I am twenty-five, and he is forty-eight. He is in a wheelchair, has been in one since 1949, and baby he has more energy than a young man when it comes down to fucking. We have a lot of fire, and believe me, we burn it all up. The days of Zip Zam Thank You Ma'am are all over with.

I really enjoyed your book.

□ One of Sherri's great frustrations is that she cannot share her fantasies with her husband: ". . . even after ten years of marriage, he still does not fully love me or trust me." So she is silent about the waking dreams that might fill their bedroom hours with life.

Sherri's letter strikes a sympathetic chord in me; she makes me sigh at the barriers within us all. They cause so much wasted happiness, so much time lost. I do not see her husband as a cold-hearted villain as much as just one more person who feels he cannot trust what he does not know. The irony is that Sherri is ready—eager—to let him know her deepest thoughts; she wishes to display herself to him in all her nakedness. It is heartbreaking to realize that his distrust will make it highly unlikely for him ever to find out what her sexual fantasies are, and to enjoy them with her.

Ginger sounds more fortunate. She reports that she is learning to use her sexual fantasies to excite her husband. She selected two of the fantasies from *My Secret Garden* and read them to him, "casually." The result delighted her—"he got a hard-on." Perhaps encouraged by this, Ginger's husband himself has begun making up fantasies. "Once," she says happily, *"my husband* made up a good airport fantasy." Her underlined words are all the evidence we need to tell us the great pleasure she felt in sharing one of his inventions.

Ricky married the only man she had ever had intercourse with, but while her husband brought home quite "a few tricks" from his time with the Navy in the South Pacific and the Orient, she finds "After a while, even the most bizarre positions become boring." Having known only one man in her life, she says she finds that "his feel, his mannerisms, are too familiar. . . . I am terribly curious if there is a noticeable difference between men. . . . I want to know so very much and plan to know no matter if I am married or not." Apparently, she has not yet found out; in the meantime, she satisfies her desire for variety in fantasies instead.

Early marriages are often disastrous; the truth is not that many people cannot lead rich lives having known only one other person sexually. The truth is that too many people do not know themselves before they marry. A woman who marries the first man she ever goes to bed with is often plagued by lifelong curiosities like Ricky's. Her letter ends on a wistful note: "I guess some people would say I was a sexually frustrated person. I love sex and touching. I feel I need sex and affection to remain emotionally and mentally healthy. . . ."

Like the remaining women in this chapter, Ricky tells us the fantasies she uses to explore as yet untasted sexual pleasures at the feast of life. □

Sherri

Thank you for *My Secret Garden*. I only wish I could speak my mind, and I wish I could share my fantasies with my husband—but even after ten years of marriage, he still does not fully love me or trust me. I enclose three of my favorite fantasies for your new book. I hope it will help other women to better understand themselves as *My Secret Garden* has helped me. My very best wishes for you and your future books.

My fantasies right now deal mainly with a couple with whom my husband and I spend a great deal of time. We are all in our early thirties, white, middle class, college educated.

My girl friend's husband is always kidding me about running off somewhere with him, or telling my husband that I'm the "prettiest girl in town" and that any man around would want to lay me if they had the chance. My husband thinks this is all a big joke, and though I've never encouraged this fellow in any way, I'm sure he'd screw me at the first opportunity if I gave him the okay. He's usually running his wife down in front of other people anyway, so she thinks that his comments to me are just another way of giving her a hard time.

On to the fantasy part:

Fantasy 1: When I masturbate (daily at least!), I sometimes imagine that my girl friend is away on business, and I've agreed to take care of her kids for her. While the kids are at school, her husband comes home. We go through the usual jokes and propositions, but this time, I know he's going to go through with it if I want him to. He pulls me close to him and starts kissing my face and throat; then as I can feel his cock come erect against my belly, he forces his tongue into my mouth. We go into the bedroom, and he takes my clothes off very slowly. He lays me over the side of the bed with my knees over the edge and starts to lick and kiss my cunt. In between licks, he's telling me how beautiful I am, that my breasts are so much larger than his wife's and that my figure is so much softer and more curved than hers. After he's licked and sucked me to the point where I'm almost exhausted, he slides me up farther on the bed and slowly puts his cock in my cunt. I imagine it to be very long and hot. He keeps sliding it in and out without putting any weight on my body, so all I feel is this long hot cock slipping up and down in my cunt. Because I've gotten so wet with my own juice, it takes little effort for his cock to slide easily around in me. Finally, he jams it in so hard that I think I'm being ripped apart, and BAMMM!!! we both finish at the same time!

Fantasy 2: I imagine that my girl friend and I are alone in either her house or mine, and we know that no one will be coming home for a long time. She asks me to help her shave the sides of her pussy so that the hair won't show outside of her bathing suit. I agree to help her, so we go into the bedroom, and while she lays on the bed with her legs apart, I start to shave her. By the time I've finished, we're both very excited over me touching her crotch. We both realize that we want to make love to one another. Then we take our clothes off and begin to kiss one another while lying very close together, face to face. I move down and start kissing and sucking on her breasts, then move lower and get between her legs. Her cunt is already starting to get wet when I push my tongue up in her.

For a long time, I lick her from her anus up to her clit, then run my tongue around her clit and kiss it or suck on it very softly. Then I start pressing harder with my tongue on her clit and stick my tongue up her cunt as far as I can. I keep this up until she comes. Then I let her rest just a moment before I lick her clit and vulva clean of her juice. After a short rest, then she goes down on me. First, she plays with my breasts, but what she really wants to do (what I want her to do!!!) is to get to my crotch. She does the same things to me that I've done to her, but she has a longer tongue than I have, so she can reach farther up into me than I did with her. She finally finishes me off by putting her top lip over my clit and her tongue up my cunt. I can feel the softness of the inside of her lip and the hardness of her teeth against my clit. After I come, she licks all my juice off of me.

Fantasy 3: (This fantasy has nothing to do with this couple.) I've traveled back in time to Imperial Japan (about AD 1500), and I'm being given to the emperor as a gift. (I don't know who's giving me away or why.) I know that the emperor has never had a white woman before, and he is very excited about me. I'm bathed, perfumed, and dressed in a beautiful kimono. Even though the kimono is heavy and completely concealing, I'm very aware that I have nothing on underneath it. When I'm brought before the emperor, everyone in the court stops talking and turns toward me. He has me stand next to him and opens my kimono so that everyone can see how beautiful my body is. He touches my hair (on my head) and then touches and strokes my pussy, because he's so taken by the sight and feel of soft blonde hair. He has attendants take me to his bedroom to await him. They remove my kimono and lay me on the bed (on the floor—Japanese style). When the emperor comes in, he sits in a low chair by my side and motions a huge, handsome guard to get me ready for him. The guard kneels between my legs and starts to lick my vulva and clit. He keeps on licking in long hot strokes and running his tongue (a very long one) up my cunt faster and faster. Now the emperor has opened his kimono, and I see that he has a huge cock that is hard and stiff as a piece of wood, and it has this beautiful soft brown tip. Even though the guard is driving me wild with his tongue up my cunt, I move over to the emperor and start to suck his cock. He doesn't try to shove it deeper into my throat, he just leans back in his chair and enjoys what I'm doing to him while he runs his hands through my long blonde hair. By now the guard is under me with his tongue up my cunt as far as he can. Just as the emperor comes and his juice shoots into my mouth, I climax from what the guard is doing to me, and push as hard as I can against his face with my crotch.

Ginger

I love your book. What a TURN-ON! I wish I could have contributed to it, but I want to tell you about myself. I married a man fifteen years my senior. For the most part, he's a codger and leaves me unsatisfied. I don't know HOW to have an orgasm. We only have sex once a week or less. He's thirty-eight; I'm twenty-three. We've been married four years. I've yearned to have affairs, but I'm not beautiful and never have found anyone who would lay me. I never asked men to, but hinted around and tried to lead them on. (It never worked.) I used to fantasize about famous men: Dick Martin, Tom Snyder. The past week, I've fantasized about the clerk in the bookstore where I bought your book. I had two encounters with him, but I don't remember him, although he said we went to the same high school. He's engaged and I want to lay him before he gets married. I feel very bad about "Nobody wants me sexually." It's such a downer with my husband's apparent lack of desire. I feel suicidal about it sometimes. Nancy, I'd screw ANYBODY!!! (or anything!)

Jim, the man I loved deeply, never asked me out when I was single (I don't like to remember that I asked him out, and he flat-out, rather tactlessly refused to go out with me). Jim is married now, and I don't think he knows how much I still love him. I've had a lot of fantasies about trying to trap Jim into fucking . . . or even just touching me. I fantasize that the next time he comes over alone I fake that I've just been assaulted in my apartment when he finds me. I'd lay there "pretending" to be "out." I'd be wearing torn-off clothing, with my legs wide open and my bare pussy peeking out. I'd be positioned with my head against something hard, with some blood on my scalp. He'd *have* to pick me up off the floor and carry me to the couch or my bed. He'd pay attention to me. Who knows, he might even fuck me! I'd "come to" after a reasonable length of time. I'd make him promise not to call the police. I'd tell him it was incest . . . like my husband's brother was the one who'd raped me. The major difference between this fantasy and the ones in your book is that I don't feel guilty about it. I'm manipulating him to the point where he can take advantage of me or not. His choice. At any rate, he'd have to touch me. That would be enough. But I'm not tied up or being forced into it. I'd do it, willingly, gladly, and guiltlessly—damn it, if anyone would only do it with me!

The other women fantasies and the dog fantasies turn me on. Once *my husband* made up a good airport fantasy: we're total strangers in the airport terminal. I'm walking along, and he's walking in back of me. I've no panties on and a short skirt, and I'm struggling with several pieces of luggage, my handbag, and sunglasses. I drop my sunglasses. He is unzipped, with his throbbing cock sticking out of his pants. I bend over from the waist to pick up what I've dropped, and he "bumps" into me. We both struggle with our luggage and fall facedown on the floor. We both screw slowly and gradually other people casually come along and join in. We rearrange ourselves face up, and we all roll around and suck and fuck each other.

In reality, I want my husband to suck and kiss and lick my cunt. He won't, willingly, only when I really pressure and nag him to do it to me. Last night, I got a hunch and acted on it. I carefully selected two of the fantasies from your book and read them to him, casually. They were "Jo" and "Wanda" (The Zoo). He got a hard-on. I want a big dog. I've fucked with a dog when I was a teenager and liked it. I think my husband would be quite stimulated to see the dog fucking me, and he'd probably mount the dog all at the same time. We live in an apartment where dogs aren't permitted, so it will be at least two years before I can get one, unless I can "borrow" one somewhere. I much thank you for caring enough to ask us for our fantasies.

How in the world are you going to top *Secret Garden?* I've been in a constant state of "moistness" since yesterday morning, when I started reading it!

Ricky

I want to write you because I enjoyed *My Secret Garden* so very much. I found it informative, interesting, entertaining, funny, shocking, and even a bit stimulating (sexually).

I fantasize. I've tried to imagine my husband as another man, but have failed. He is the only man I have ever had intercourse with, and after three years of simply one man, I have found that his feel, his mannerisms, are too familiar to get into my head that he is another man.

I do daydream about sex. I am terribly curious if there is a noticeable difference between men. Can you tell the difference in their size just from the feel of their organ deep (or not so deep) inside that warm, soft spot? Are their "styles" noticeably different? I want to know so very much and plan to know no matter if I am married or not.

My hubsand was in the Navy when we met and started to sleep together. (There was no "sleeping" until we were married though.) He brought home from the South Pacific and the Orient a few tricks. He showed me so many positions that I can't number them nor do I care to. After a while, even the most bizarre positions become boring. The day we were married, he lost a great deal of interest in sex. He says that there was a great deal of "challenge" before we were married. Now it is here anytime he wants it. He turns to me when he feels the urge, not the deep beauty of it, but the natural call of his sexual drive. About eight to fourteen days apart and never more than once a night. He is always ready for me to give him head though. Not to have sex or eat me when I feel like it.

My daydreams are of men I have met. I imagine we are alone, and he tenderly, slowly makes love to me. No, I make love to him right back. He shows that he really enjoys what I do to and with him. He moves about, he makes low, sexy noises, he holds me tighter. (My husband is a quiet man, never makes a sound. He claims to have only one "hot spot"—his dick.) We give and take from each other in the most beautiful act in creation. So far I have not been able to set an end to this fantasy. I sometimes have a climax during it, but that isn't all too important to me. (I always enjoy foreplay the most.)

Sometimes the man is famous. My idol is Joe Namath. Sometimes he is a man I have met casually; sometimes he is a friend of my husband's. My husband knows that

I have a sexual attraction to this *one* friend of his. It came out in a "What if" conversation. He knows and I believe myself when I say I doubt if I could carry through with an affair. It would take an advance from the man. A subtle one, a tender one.

I feel I wouldn't be honest if I didn't tell you that I do have this "daydream" about my half-brother. We have the same father. Both our mothers were divorced from our father, and we seldom saw each other in sixteen years. He finally became closer and closer to our father. (I always was, though not sexually attracted to our father.) We began seeing each other and writing. Since we did not have a chance to develop a brother-sister relationship, I do not feel that way toward him. I feel at times that he does not regard me as a "sister." He is a tender person, and I sometimes feel he would like to ball me as I would him. The fact that we have the same father seems to stop us both. I know if he would let me know or make a move, I would jump. I am not afraid to be the instigator in sex. I just need to know the man I'm interested in is interested in me. He comes on (my brother) as a very sensual person. He belongs to a nudist camp in the hills. He is also a very sensual photographer. Soft, moody, beautiful works. (Our father is a photographer; he is a part-time pro.)

I guess some people would say I was a sexually frustrated person. I have been told I am a sexual person. I love sex and touching. I feel I need sex and affection to remain emotionally and mentally healthy. I hope you can use this. Please let me know what you think.

Stella

I just finished reading your book and found it very exciting, to say the least. I told a couple of my friends about it, and am sorry to say that they aren't open-minded enough to read it too.

My sex life started at the age of twenty-one at my own request. I used to very often sleep with this one guy with the usual foreplay, but when it got to "the limit," *nothing more*. Being a romantic-type person, I asked him one night to make love to me. The conclusion, unfortunately, was the question to myself: Is that all there is?

Since then, there have been a few more men, but all I seem to be doing is running into the same kind of people. They satisfy themselves and leave me very frustrated and still waiting for something to happen.

I love sex, to say the least, and never have regretted having given up my womanly treasure, so to speak. I am now twenty-five and have lived with a guy three years. Our sex life is very dull, maybe because I just don't try. But *he* just doesn't do anything for me sexually.

Why I stay is another story in itself. I have had other flings since this guy I live with, but never seem to find satisfaction. I'm trying to find out what a climax is all about!

Thinking back over your book, I found myself in there a number of times. If I were to tell you my fantasies, they would be much like many other women's. What I find sex is all about is people together, sharing, feeling, caring. I often wonder what a certain person would be like. I see a man at the office or at a party, and I try to imagine what it would be like to make love to him. But I'm always afraid my dreams will end up like my reality—better in the imagination than in the performance. So many men think that just because they've reached a climax, the woman must have been satisfied too. I suppose I will keep looking for a man who does not believe this, who understands women better. But in the meantime, I suppose I must just stick to my dreams.

Jill

A friend of mine recently recommended your book to me, so I bought a copy. I have just finished reading it. I saw on a back page a request for suggestions, comments, and further fantasies, and that is why I am writing to you. I think your book is great. Until now, I have always thought that my fantasies were something bad that I should keep hidden. I was afraid that there was something wrong with me, because I often had these "bad" sexual fantasies, and because I enjoyed them. It relieves some of my fears to know that other women have sexual fantasies just as I do.

I would like to share some of my fantasies with you, and maybe they will help you in preparing your second book. Let me tell you something about myself first. I used to work as a secretary, but now I am just a housewife. I spend most of my time at home and since I have no children, I get very bored and lonely. My husband has the kind of job in which he has no set work hours. He often comes home very late, and then he brings work home with him. He often has to work on weekends too. I really think that we were together more before we were married. Even when I go to bed at night, he is usually still up doing some work he brought home. He never seems to have time for me anymore. He seldom has time for sex either. Even when I come right out and ask him to make love to me, he usually says that he is too busy or that he does not have any time to waste. When he does make love to me, he acts like it is some kind of routine thing, like brushing his teeth or shaving. He acts like he is in a hurry to get it done. Lately, he has been telling me that he does not have time to make love to me, but that he will masturbate me for a little while if I want him to. He often tells me that I should learn to control my sexual feelings and that there are more important things in life than sex. Because my real sexual life is not what I want it to be, I have had to fantasize a good sexual life for myself. I spend much of the time that I am home alone fantasizing and masturbating. I have developed a whole collection of fantasies, and I would like to share some of them with you.

In my favorite fantasy, I see myself as a Near Eastern ruler like those long ago. I live in a "pleasure palace" with a whole "harem" of men. They are always available to satisfy whatever sexual desires I have. In my mind, I have them categorized in a kind of filing system. Each man is categorized according to his age, his looks and physical build, his sexual skills (that is, the sexual skills I imagine he has), and his general personality. Most of the men in my harem are men I know or have known, but some are imaginary men, or men I know about but do not really know personally. In the sexual skills category, I classify each man according to his general skill at lovemaking, his powers of endurance during lovemaking, his skill at oral lovemaking, and any other sexual skills he has. I also rate each man in my harem according to the size of his penis, his ability to use it, and whether or not it is circumcised. I like variety, so these men are all different from each other. I can select one according to what I am looking for at the time.

In a typical fantasy of this kind, I am in a large, opulent bedroom in my "pleasure palace." I am usually dressed in a sensual, silky nightgown. In the bedroom, there is a huge canopy bed upon which I am lying. As I try to decide which man (or men) I want, I lie there masturbating, both in my fantasy and in reality. When I select the man I want, he is brought to my bedroom. As I watch, he is taken to an adjoining bathroom where my servants (all female) undress him and bathe him. When they have dried him and put cologne on him, my servants bring him to my bed, and then they leave the room. The man I have selected wants very much to make love to me, but I make him stand at the side of my bed and wait until I am ready. Often at this point, I get out of bed and undress while he watches. He must stand at attention and not move while I entice him. When I am nude, I come over to him and caress him and rub my body against him, but he must remain at attention. When I have teased him enough, I lie down on the bed and allow him to lie down with me and make love to me. If I desire oral lovemaking, I lie with my legs over the side of the bed, and he kneels beside the bed and makes love to me orally. Other times, I sit on the edge of the bed or kneel and make him stand right in front of me. Then I make love to him orally. In fantasies in which I make love to him orally, I usually imagine that his penis is still soft and that it swells and becomes erect in my mouth. As I said, the men are different, so the kind of lovemaking that I have with each one is different. All of them are very passionate though. Usually, I make love for a long time with the man I select. He is able to delay his orgasm until the end, or he is able to have more than one orgasm. All of the men in my fantasies are able to do one of these two things. That may be because my husband can do neither one of them, and I wish he could. In my fantasies, the men I choose and I make love in many different positions. That, too, is different from making love with my husband, because he always insists on using the same position, the standard one with him on top.

This kind of fantasy lets me imagine an unlimited number of variations of it. One of my favorite variations of it is one in which my husband is humiliated and made to suffer. In this fantasy, my husband is the man who is brought to my bedroom. When my servants undress him and bathe him, they make fun of him and laugh at him. Most of all, they tease him about the small size of his penis. They tell him his penis looks like a little boy's. In reality, it does look more like a boy's than a man's. He is very self-conscious about the small size of his penis, and he often asks me if it bothers me that his penis is so small. I always tell him that it does not bother me, but sometimes I would like to tell him what I really think. In this fantasy, my servants tease him by telling him some of the things about his small penis that I would often like to tell him. When my servants bring him to my bed, they stay and watch instead of leaving. He pleads for me to undress and make love with him, but I refuse. Still dressed in my gown, I stand close to him and whisper in his ear about all the pleasures he would feel if he made love with me. He gets very excited and gets an erection, and he cannot wait any longer. He takes a hold of his penis to masturbate himself, but the moment he touches it, he ejaculates. My servants, who are watching, laugh at him and tease him. They call him "the fastest gun of all." He is very ashamed and embarrassed, and he pleads with me to give him another chance. I refuse, and I tell him that he will see how a real man makes love with a woman. Then I order my servants to tie him to a pillar so that he is facing my bed.

With my husband there watching, I have one of my favorite men brought to my bedroom. He is always someone whom my husband knows. Often he is a former boyfriend of mine with whom I had intercourse for the first time in my life. My husband is facing so that he can see my servants undress and bathe this man, and my husband sees that the man I have selected has a much larger penis than he does. This man's penis is as much larger than normal as my husband's is smaller than normal, and this was true about my former boyfriend whom I have just mentioned. While my husband watches, the man is brought over to my bed. I undress quickly, and kneel beside the bed so that he is right in front of me. Then I bend forward and kiss the tip of his penis. It is still soft, and I take a hold of it with my fingertips. It feels heavy. I pull back the foreskin of his penis and lick its soft, pink glans. Out of the corner of my eye, I can see my husband watching me. This man's penis is so large that I cannot get very much of it into my mouth, but I take as much of it into my mouth as I can. During the time that I have been sucking on it and licking it, it has become erect. After a few minutes of this, I stop and get back on the bed, and I invite this man to lie down with me. We slowly begin to make love. He is a very skilled lover, and he does everything that pleases me. Although he is passionate and very excited, he is not in a hurry. When I am ready, I have him lie on his back, and I get on top of him. I guide his penis into me, and it fills me completely. We go slowly at first, and we move in a way that causes his penis to make long, slow strokes in and out of me. I have several orgasms, and he is able to delay his orgasm as long as I want him to. Finally, I am ready to finish, and we go wild. Together we reach a tremendous orgasm. We lie together quietly for a few minutes, and then we are ready to start again. He still has an erection. This time, I get on my hands and knees, and he kneels in back of me and enters me from behind. Again we start slowly, and he reaches around me and caresses me with his fingers. In a while, we lose control of ourselves, and he is moving like a wild stallion. Together we reach another tremendous orgasm. Sometimes we go on and make love some more in other positions, but often it stops here. My lover and I bathe together while my husband watches. Then he dresses and returns to the harem, and my husband is left tied to the pillar. I go back to bed and lie down, and my servants tease my husband about what a poor lover he is compared to the man he has just seen. Then my husband is returned to the harem, where the other men tease him too.

I have another version of this fantasy in which a young boy is brought to my bedroom after my husband's failure. The boy has never made love to a woman before, and I teach him the right way to make love. What makes it better is that this young boy has a penis that is larger than my husband's. That really humiliates my husband. This boy learns quickly and becomes a much better lover than my husband.

I have other fantasies too. I love to fantasize about couples I know. I enjoy trying to imagine them making love. Now that several magazines for women are publishing photographs of nude men, I have found that I can become very aroused by looking at such photographs. I often look at these photographs while I am masturbating, and I fantasize about the men in them. I imagine them making love with me. I do not have fantasies in which I take part in lesbian lovemaking, but I do have fantasies in which I secretly see two other women making love. I especially enjoy fantasies in which I secretly see other people making love with each other.

I definitely do enjoy my fantasy sexual life more than my real sexual life. I think that that is the main reason why I have felt that my sexual fantasies are bad. I also have felt bad about the amount of time that I have spent fantasizing. I often spend hours at a time fantasizing and masturbating. It is the way in which I fill much of the time in which I have little else to do. Most of my fantasies are those based upon the format of my having a harem of men. I can have any man I want, and I can do whatever I want with them. I have not made any of my fantasies a reality, but, as time goes by, I feel more and more like doing so. One of these days, if the right situation arises, I may not resist the temptation to really live one of my fantasies. With the way that my husband has treated me and is treating me in regard to sex, I almost feel that I have the right to obtain sexual satisfaction where I can. I find myself looking for the right situation in which I can safely have an affair with another man. It may not be long before I find the situation that I am looking for, and then I may make some of my fantasies realities. I sometimes wonder if my husband would even care if I was having an affair with another man as long as it did not cause him any trouble. He might even like it if I would stop bothering him about sex. After all of this, though, I have to say that most of all I would prefer that my husband become a better and more satisfying lover so that all of these other things would be unnecessary. I guess that that is my biggest fantasy.

PART TWO

THE USES
OF
SEXUAL FANTASY

CHAPTER FIVE

DAYDREAMING

☐ Life can be seen as an effort toward equilibrium. If we are hungry, we eat. Tired? We rest. If we've been using our minds too strenuously, we long for physical exercise or a walk in the woods. This is also true of our inner selves . . . although many of our mental efforts at maintaining equilibrium hover on the border of unconsciousness. Daydreaming—while going about the ordinary chores of the day—is one of these activities.

Usually, our daydreams pass out of our mind without leaving a trace behind. A chance question from a neighbor, the ringing of a telephone—and suddenly we are focused on the here and now, the large part of our idle reveries forgotten. Unlike unconscious fantasies, however, it is usually not too difficult to resummon and examine our daydreams. If we do, they can tell us a lot about who we are and what is missing from our lives. This is most obviously true in the Walter Mitty kind of daydream indulged in by the average-man-lost-in-the-crowd. In his reveries, the most overblown ambitions come true. The unusual thing about sexual daydreaming is that the daydreams do not often come to women who have no sex at all. When repression is that total, sexual daydreaming is pushed underground too. Much more often, I find that women's erotic daydreams are not so much about sex itself but are about a kind of sex they have not had, or will not allow themselves. It is the effort of their imagination to supply something that is missing from their real lives.

I bridle when people try to dismiss daydreams as unimportant because they are "unreal." They are just as real as the experience of reading a novel, listening to music, or looking at paintings. They are all efforts of the mind to present us with a more satisfying order of reality, a beauty we might otherwise never have known. Jane Eyre never existed in the real world, but I am the richer for Charlotte Brontë's story about her. (After all, couldn't a novel itself be described as a disciplined daydream?)

Ordinarily, our daydreams of happiness are abruptly followed by feelings of disappointment and/or guilt. The pendulum is swinging back toward equilibrium, but goes right through the median point of stasis. We overreact; it is as if we cannot find a balance again until we have paid with mental rue and regret for the fantasized pleasures we have just pictured for ourselves. Talking about the anxieties aroused in us by our imagined actions or delights, Dr. Erik Erikson (*Childhood and Society*) says, ". . . our irrational worry . . . our fear of having aroused actually quite disinterested, and antagonized quite well-meaning people, our fantasized atonements and childish repetitions, may well surprise us."

The barriers to our happiness, the limits we allow ourselves, are more often within ourselves than outside. For fear that the man we love may think badly of us, we hesitate to ask him for simple sexual pleasures we have every right to. In our own minds, we change him from a lover to a critic . . . even worse, we make him a critic so harsh that *we know in advance* he will disapprove. Therefore, we avoid the test of reality and never ask him, never give him a chance to show us how much he himself might welcome our requests for as yet untasted pleasures. It is our own unnecessarily strict, even sadistic, consciences that keep us from sexual pleasure we have every right to enjoy.

In her very romantic letter, Lulu describes an event that she could not allow herself to have, even though the time, the place, and even the man were "right." She entitles her fantasy, "An Ideal Sexual Encounter." But at the peak of the event in real life, "my automatic 'No, thank you' intruded. . . . Were I to have enough courage, I would have whispered a simple 'Yes, I want to.' "

Lulu's letter then goes on to describe a simple daydream of happiness. While she may regret that she denied herself the fulfillment of this experience for the rest of her life, in her daydream it is hers after all. An effort of the imagination has repaired the torn fabric of the past. □

Lulu

I enjoyed your book and found the honest exposure of sexual impulse very freeing and enlightening myself.

As you can see, I was quite reserved and conflicted prior to becoming married, but the impulse and fantasies were very much alive.

P.S. I am thirty-two, married for the second time, and *very happy*. I have a master's degree and am employed full time in my profession. No children are planned in our future.

An Ideal Sexual Encounter

In truth, my ideal encounter is the cherished memory of my second date with my husband. We met at church, purely by accident, and I was immediately repelled by his frankly sexual look at me—in church, no less. Our first date was a disaster. He invited me to go sailing. I refused unless other persons were to be present for fear of being "trapped" alone with this hairy-chested male. My preoccupation was clear. A slight innuendo at sexual encounter casually made, and again I was thoroughly upset. . . I realize now I was reacting too intensely for it to be genuine protest.

My fascination with him grew, as I saw him now and

then around church and again at a party at which he was thoroughly charming, funny, and very interesting. His casual arm around my waist and a whispered, "Stay here with me," sent me scurrying into a kitchen full of gossiping women.

After agonizing months of watching him at church, I forced myself to speak to him first (a brave step forward for me), and he asked if I'd like to go for a hike to a wooded area soon to be destroyed by installation of a highway. Terrified, and delighted, I agreed. We had a pleasant walk through the woods to a waterfall, he handling my anxiety by easily chatting about his many varied and amusing experiences on his world travels. I was uneasy about even holding his hand over rough terrain. Needless to say, I was struggling with my own sexual attraction to him which I couldn't control.

Bravely, I ventured forth that I'd like to see his pictures sometime, to which he suggested that same evening would be fine. We arrived at his neat, comfortable, masculine duplex in a quiet, wooded area overlooking the lake. I was immediately impressed with his tasteful accommodations, but also with the fascinating portrait of a beautiful woman on the living-room wall—her hair loose, eyes shut, and head thrown back in an ecstasy of pleasure—clearly at the peak of orgasm. I felt helpless—caught alone with this male in a web I had woven for myself. I wanted to go home. The other side of me decided within minutes after arrival that I wanted to live here forever with this man whom I really didn't even know.

Tony flicked on the radio to a quiet station and in the darkening evening built an intimate fire for two. The enormous sofa, spread with a soft alpaca coverlet (picked up on a recent trip to Peru), was pushed close to the raised hearth on which he spread cheeses, crackers, marinated mushrooms, and two glasses of scotch. The wooden bases were intricately carved mahogany which he had created himself. Then he returned to a bright kitchen to prepare dinner. I stared into the fire trying to recover my composure. The portrait of the woman seemed to be mocking me. . . .

Shortly thereafter, Tony settled on the sofa, cheerfully announcing dinner would be ready in about two hours. His special spaghetti sauce requires that long to simmer. Inwardly gasping at such a long period of unstructured time, I asked if he were going to show me his pictures.

He did. The pictures were vivid and intriguing scenes of the ancient Incan ruins of Machu Picchu, Peru. In contrast to this presentation, he showed fantastic pictures of Antarctica: icebergs, roaring seas, glorious sunsets, and his work and colleagues' on board ship. I was enchanted with this all-male domain in an environment I saw was as rugged and as naturally beautiful as the men themselves.

Dinner was served at the hearth: spaghetti, salad, red wine, and I was getting tipsy. Afterward, he snuggled close, and we kissed. I loved it. Tony is a superb kisser, passionate and yet tender. Rubbing over my body with his hands, he talked of how much he enjoyed sex, enjoyed active women, and liked to kiss their genitals. He mentioned his previous wife did not like her clitoris touched. I clinically offered she had childhood prohibitions against masturbation. He visibly brightened and happily remarked he was so glad that I "did it." I vanished behind my professional mask and told him I was discussing *her*, not *me!* Tony looked puzzled and said *he* was discussing *me*.

We kissed often and longer that evening, me getting extremely slippery and hotter and hotter. Tony's erect thrusting penis felt so good against my pubic area—it had been so long since I'd been with a man!! I was as famished for sex as for the meal he served.

Tony's body was becoming hot also, and he began to sweat and took off his shirt. I lightly caressed and rubbed his back and, out of irresistible curiosity, softly reached around to touch the mass of delicious hair on his chest, exploring until I accidently (?) touched his erect nipple. He whispered, "You can stay here all night if you want to."

[My encounter is true to this point. My automatic "No, thank you" intruded here, even though he later showed me his bedroom, complete with huge waterbed, fluffy down-filled comforter (from long unheated winter nights in Europe), heat lamps over the bed for comfort, and another "delight" I later learned to enjoy was a vibrator. I did want to stay!]

Were I to have enough courage, I would have whispered a simple "Yes, I want to." I would have undressed him, pulling off his belt, spanking his buttocks playfully and briefly with it, untying his shoes, slipping off his socks, very slowly unzipping and dropping his trousers, letting them tickle his inner thighs as they went down. Then I would remove my top, shoes, and slacks to black lace bra and black lace bikini panties. In the firelight, with him standing, I would slowly pull off his underwear, letting the elastic tickle his stomach; and when his enormous, engorged, erect penis burst forth, I would kiss it gently and tenderly up and down the shaft, cradling his balls, gently pulling on both occasionally. Then I would lick the ticklish spot underneath, around the tip, caressing the "eye" with my tongue. He begins pushing toward me, and I allow it in my mouth, sucking and swallowing as much as possible. Tony moves to and fro in spasms of pleasure. . . .

Tony lets down my long hair and buries his face in it, kissing my neck. He quickly pulls off my panties, undoes my bra, admiring my figure in the firelight, running his hands lightly across breasts, stopping to pull and knead them, then quickly on to belly and teasingly up the vaginal crack, allowing his finger to slightly touch and tease the vagina and deliciously tickling my clitoris in passing. An intimate tongue in the vagina and more delicious tickling the clitoris with his tongue, and he picks me up, carrying me to his bed, which is already warm from the heat lamps.

Intercourse begins. I am frantic for the weight of him,

for the determined shove of his member into my warm waiting body, pouring forth water as the falls we had seen that afternoon. With groans of pleasure, he begins thrusting deep, pressing the cervix, each of us releasing pent-up emotion that only the single (or I) can accumulate. I, sweating and crying, respond to his passion with clutching hands, heaving hips, back arched in anticipation, and burning pleasure in my cunt. My mind runs over and over the thought, "Fuck me, Tony, fuck me." And then it goes blank. . . .

I am torn between the fear of the animal passions released and desperate desire for the raging fire spreading over me. I have no choice now. Tony's urgent thrusts are my own, and together we are both driven madly toward the final shattering moments when we surrender to our lust. Gasping, arching, I am consumed in Tony's manliness and exist alone no more. I have no words to express my feelings at our union, only cries from my shattered soul.

Sobbing into Tony's neck and shoulder, I regain consciousness. He holds me tenderly, kissing my neck, rocking me slightly. I feel tremendous relief and gratitude toward him. I am floating with joy. He is mine, and I am his. A tiny fire burns within me still which he caresses with his fingers to full flame. I have a series of minor orgasms, only reflections of our first passion. Grateful and exhausted, I fall asleep in his encircling arms. . .

☐ We are all used to seeing magazine advertisements or television commercials of a woman daydreaming at the window or while looking into a fireplace. If a man lost in an idle reverie of pipe smoke were asked what dreams he sees suspended before his eyes, he might well laugh and say, "Sophia Loren, who wants to seduce me." But a woman is taught, by these exercises of salesmanship, that *her* correct answer is that she is dreaming of a whiter laundry than her neighbors, or finding a baby food that will make her child grow six feet tall. We are not allowed the uses of erotic reverie that reinforce us in our own minds as sexual beings. No wonder so many women who can think of themselves only in the role of Mrs. Superconsumer, resist seeing themselves in any image that smacks of eroticism.

Fernando Sanchez is the designer of some of the most feminine, beautiful lingerie in America today. They are truly the stuff of which a woman's most sensuous dreams can be made . . . lovingly cut peignoirs with panels of lace . . . negligees that entrance the beholder with the grace and erotic promise of the female body. And yet Mr. Sanchez recently told me, "Our big problem is to educate women to seeing themselves in seductive clothes like these. They may stop and admire a tempting nightgown on a model in a store, or in a fashion magazine, but even in these liberated times, the woman will usually just sigh and say, 'That's not me,' and head for the drip dry counter." But if she's not an erotic woman, who is she?

One letter from a woman named Cheryl is an example of how women are conditioned to fight their own sexuality. She was so inhibited in her own mind that she never once climaxed during the three years she lived on and off with a man to whom she was engaged. "Before him," she says, "I was a virgin and tried masturbation." But even that did not work for her. Defeated, she writes forlornly, "I gave up trying."

It was only recently, at the age of twenty-four, that she met a new young man and "could finally relax completely, enjoying my new freedom, and I 'came' for the first time ever." As if to further underline the distance she had been taught to keep between herself and her own sexuality, she says she wasn't even certain she had experienced orgasm with this new man—or at least, didn't "realize it fully until a short time ago."

One of the healthiest aspects of human nature is that it does fight for equilibrium; once repression has been lifted, it can work with the speed of a coiled spring to right the balance. Now that Cheryl accepts her sexual self, her old bugaboos seem to be vanishing. I find her closing very moving: her new sexual self-confidence, she says, has made her "very proud of myself. . . ." She feels she is a woman at last.

In her letter, Jackie also writes that facing her own sexuality frankly has been an important step forward in life. She writes that she and her older brother used to play sexual games as children. This is hardly unusual for young siblings; nevertheless, she found these activities so disturbing that "I used to hide my head under the pillow to make the reality of the responsibility 'go away.' "

If Jackie disavowed her sexual experience by hiding her head under the pillow, another form of denial is to have sexual events take place as if you yourself were just a spectator. It's not happening to you, but to somebody else. In Samantha's poetic fantasy, which she calls "The Blue Star," this is exactly what happens. The entire fantasy is told third person, as if it had no relation to Samantha at all.

It is easy to see that this method of sexual fantasy is a strategy for avoiding guilt; it is a daydream about having the most marvelous sexual experience—but experiencing the whole thing vicariously in the third person.

In Connie's fantasy too, the same emotions seem to be the basis for the sexual scenario she invents. "Faceless, hooded, sexless people are tightening straps to my wrists and ankles," she writes, describing the circumstances of her favorite fantasy, in which she enjoys sex without responsibility, without choice.

These sexual fantasies, which seek to combine the maximum of erotic arousal and satisfaction with the minimum of guilt, reach their logical conclusion in fantasies in which the woman is given absolutely no choice in the matter at all . . . fantasies of force or rape. "The doorbell rings," Elaine writes of one such fantasy. "A good-looking young man pushes his way in, grabs me. . . ." The sexual act takes place, but it is not the woman's fault. She "did not ask for it."

What we must remember is that for most women, who have never experienced rape, the word just represents an abstract idea; combining rape with sex in their fantasies is just *using* rape, almost as a theatrical convention—it is a means toward an end. When understood this way, rape becomes code language for, "It wasn't my fault," or just as simply, "He wanted me so much, he overpowered me. You can't blame me if I am such an overwhelmngly sexually attractive creature that I drove him mad with lust *despite all I could do to fight him off!*"

If the women who fantasize about rape were really turned on by the ugliness and brutality of it, in their imagined scenarios they would describe the feelings of disgust, shame, and degradation ensuing from this physiological and psychological assault. But on the contrary! When you read these rape fantasies, which, after all, have been entirely created by the women concerned for their own pleasure, the elements of force and brutality are seen to be not important at all. What happens instead is that the force and ardor of their rapist-lover allows them to release all their own pent-up sexual force, power. Every thrust of his powerful hand, forcing them down, is returned by a thrust of their own—which can be read as protest, but which is clearly a sexual release on the woman's part, as guiltless as it is powerful. The man's demands on her body are the demands of a lust she has always been too inhibited to respond to with all the sexual force and vibrancy of her own body; fantasy allows her to respond at last like some kind of sexual animal to his animal treatment—a most unladylike way to behave, even unwomanly, unless you can mask your "aggressive" actions as protest.

If the women in these rape fantasies were concerned with the pain of rape, if they even elaborated on the pain involved, the fantasies could be called masochistic. But these aren't fantasies about the pleasure of pain. They are imaginary scenarios speaking of a romantic desire for unromantic sex: these women don't want love (at least this one time) in a bower of flowers in a tender lover's arms. They want sweat, roll-around, knock-about thrust-and-counterthrust, with no holds barred. They want sex that transcends any limits they have ever known with a man who won't take less than a woman is capable of giving. And most women are capable of giving a hell of a lot more sexual thrust and emotion than they think most men want, or that they themselves are capable of (being "nice" women). The fantasy of rape solves all these problems, provides all this pleasure. Rape? These women don't want rape. They want release.

But before we leave this subject, let me add one very strong proviso: we must be clear that enjoying an emotion in fantasy does not necessarily mean you want to live it out in reality. If you become angry, for instance, you might say to someone, "If you do that again, I'll kill you!" The words may even be accompanied by a very satisfying quick image of the offender lying dead at your feet. But no one—least of all you—really believes that these fantasies of violence are ideas that you have any intention of carrying out. You just wanted the momentary release of *expressing* strong emotion, but only in words, merely as an idea. Fantasies from women like Jackie, Samantha, Connie, Elaine . . . fantasies of being sexually forced or raped . . . are in the same category: they may be satisfying to think about, they give the woman license, at least in her imagination, to enjoy herself sexually, and they remove her from any feeling of guilt, because she never had any choice in the matter—but there isn't a woman I know who wouldn't run a mile if she thought there was the slightest chance it would happen in real life.

There is a safety in fantasy. In our minds, we can test certain situations to see how they might feel; we always know that no matter how sordid the emotions we are dealing with, no matter how angry, gigantic, or demanding the characters, they are all puppets of our own invention. If any of these ideas ever become too frightening, we can turn them off like turning the pages of a book. This, I believe, is the final ingredient in the glamor that rape holds in some fantasies. In the safe playground of our minds, we can toy with the male's most dangerous, most aroused emotions—and use them for just the whim and fancy of our idle moment. He may be raging, threatening, or even hurting us in the fantasy, *but in reality we control him!* ☐

Jackie

Throughout the reading of your *Secret Garden,* I was wavering between hope and fear that at the end you would (not) request more fantasies. Reading of other women, I found myself wishing you had a group going where I could tell everyone mine.

I am twenty-nine, never married, highly intelligent (150 IQ) well educated, and overwhelmingly fat and frustrated. I did not discover myself, as some of your contributors state, but at the age of five my brother discovered me. We were hiding in a clothes closet, and he pulled down my panties and explored me with a flashlight—giggling excitedly and urging me to be quiet. I was afraid of my brother even then, and was—although I did not understand it—horribly humiliated. After that, I became curious about myself and would masturbate. My mother effectively made me feel guilty about this: each morning, she would smell my hands and say, "Your hands smell like they've been in the wrong place." She couldn't, however, stop me—or my brother.

One of my earliest fantasies occurred when I was four years old and would sleep on my parents' bed until their bedtime. I would dream that a doctor came in to give me an injection. I remember screaming in my fantasy for my mother, but she would not save me. It was a terribly exciting idea, this fearsome happening. Perhaps this sexual preoccupation stems from my brother or from the fact that I slept in my parents' bedroom until I was five.

My brother and I played many sexual games—doctor and actress, doctor and patient, husband and wife, and we had ample opportunity, since both my parents worked. When they were around, we would fight and hate each other. One disturbing aspect (to me it still is) is that we never kissed or spoke to each other. I used to hide my head under the pillow to make the reality of the responsibility "go away." My brother is four years older than I and was always stronger. When we fought, he hurt me (am I rationalizing?). I mentally refused to accept any responsibility for our acts. We continued until I was eighteen, and he got married. I was very upset and depressed about his marriage—but couldn't fathom why. In fact, I never understood this whole thing until I went into analysis.

Since he married, I had other men, but never have an orgasm (we never had one when we were kids either). Each case is similar: I always feel horribly humiliated and hate myself afterward. I have never really been in love. I can't achieve orgasm even when I masturbate.

My fantasies as a child were usually about doctors telling me what a brave little girl I am while they "examined" me sexually. Usually in groups of three or four. I have once or twice "caught" myself having a lesbian fantasy, but stopped because I was afraid it would make me a lesbian. I say "was" because since I've read your book, I can see that it is not freakish, and I feel more free. I can't thank you enough for publishing your book.

As I grew older, my fantasies about doctors ceased, and I remember really getting turned on at college lectures by just imagining myself screwing with the professor. Later, I had fantasies about my analyst, though not really sexual. Mostly, I wanted to be a little bird that could nest in the hair in his armpits. I used to despise women, but that is changing now. I find I have more respect for other women . . . but only if they are intelligent. I'm still seeking a meaningful relationship with a man, and I'm not afraid anymore. In truth, I think I was afraid that both men and women only wanted to use me, hurt me, and degrade me. Knowing my sexual fantasies has helped me to reach my new self-acceptance. Your book has made me feel so much better about myself. Thank you.

Ethel

I too thought I was crazy, because I had these fantasies, but now I know it is normal, because I read your book. I am no lesbian, but I have thought a number of times about this particular fantasy. I would daydream that a man with a knife would knock on my door, and when I opened it, push me in and then tell his two women to come in. He would tie me up, and then the two women would undress me. One is black, and one is white. The black woman has a whip and is naked with only black boots on. She would tie me to the bed, and then the white one would spread my legs, and the black one would get on me and start eating me out. When finished, the black one would get off and sit on my face so I could eat her, while the white one inserted a vibrator into my cunt. After a while, she takes it out and tongue fucks me and after a while would place her finger in my juicy wet cunt up and down till I had an orgasm. The man would be masturbating while watching. After this, they would all tie my legs up strongly, and the white girl would open my mouth while the man let me blow him and the black chick is fingering me. Wow, I'm horny now. I have more to tell, but it would take a book. Thanks for letting me talk.

P.S. Believe me this is no joke. I am only eighteen with one boy aged two, and a husband aged thirty-two.

Samantha

The Blue Star

The room was guarded by statues of marble, shadowy figures in the outer halls. The silence was penetrated slightly by eerie music, unearthly in form.

Inside the huge doors, carved by a sculptor's patient hand seemingly, lay a magnificent room. It had a cathedral quality—high vaulted ceiling, ornate gilded walls, immaculate stone floor. And at the very peak of the room, the ceiling's center, there was a glorious, thick, glass Star of David. The sapphire blue was almost smoky, but light played through in drifting waves.

The girl lay underneath on a long, ceremonial table, tied hand, foot to the four corners of the rather wide rectangle. She was naked save for a wooden crucifix around her neck. She lay meditatively intent upon the pulsating star in the center of her vision. At times, she almost luxuriously strained her limbs against the coils of rope on her wrists and ankles. But her gaze never changed. Nor her expression. She lay hypnotized by the glazed star; it burned her eyes and heart.

Silently, four rows of men took their places around the table. She felt their presence intimately like a stabbing wound. They were dressed in simple garb, a long robe of sackcloth knotted with a length of rope. They began a chant, low and soft and pure, that made her feel strong, almost pure, highly exalted. The light was dimmer now. She flicked her tongue over her lips, feeling warm moisture fill the cleft between her legs. Her nipples began to harden, and as though this were a new experience, she began to softly groan, her eyes still fixed on the blue star above her head. The chant grew louder.

One of the monks took his place at the table's end. He touched the soft white feet delicately, then climbed on her full length. He kissed the small red mouth and lay still. The harsh sackcloth rubbed against her, stinging the fair skin, but as his erection grew, she lost herself to the feel of his hard manhood against her stomach. He rolled aside suddenly and removed the garment. She turned her head slowly and saw him, a tall and strong David, white and ruddy. He had dark, curly hair that curled around his erect penis as well. He looked at her kindly as he sensed her amazement at its size. She began to feel long-denied urges penetrate her to the core, strange and drifting blue.

The man climbed on her again, kissing her from her feet to her willing hungry mouth. The men began their low chant again. As they did, he inserted his penis into her. It reminded her vaguely of a knife being put into its sheath.

After a long, sweet love, they all took their turns caressing her from head to foot, moaning and chanting and filling her with their love.

And as she drifted off, weary and complete, the face of the first David filled her mind. The star filled her eyes, and a drowsy lassitude, her body. She fell asleep.

Debbie

I am seventeen and have been screwing for over two years. My lovers have ranged from nineteen to thirty-four, although I prefer the older men. I am very experienced and very good—and I know it. I have had many affairs with married men and have loved every minute.

I had had fantasies ever since I was in the fifth grade. The fantasies I had up till the eighth grade involved my male teachers. My freshman year, I began screwing around. It was extremely painful the first couple of times, and I never was satisfied, but I knew there had to be something terrific about sex, so I kept at it until I was one of the hottest numbers around.

My fantasies lately have involved me driving in a

mountainous area. My car goes into a skid and I crash. A gorgeous man finds me. He feels instant compassion for me. I'm in a strange town, so the man decides to look out for me. The climax of the story comes on a dark stormy night. I am living in his house. It is thundering very loudly, and I am frightened. There is a knock at my bedroom door. I clutch my flimsy nightgown to me. He walks in and looks at me and tries to act cool. He has come to find out if I'm all right. I sit on the bed with my legs tucked under me. I reach for something, and my legs spread apart. (I have no underwear on, of course.) His eyes never leave me. Our eyes meet for a long look. I call his name, and he sits on the bed beside me. He kisses me, his tongue going deeply, and he fondles my tits. He parts my nightgown and his tongue caresses me everywhere until finally he comes to my clitoris on which he concentrates all his efforts. All the while, he finger fucks me in my vagina and anus (which I love) until I climax. After this, I take out his cock and lick and suck his cock and balls.

One other fantasy I have is being raped by six or more men. One frenching me, one on each tit, caressing and licking it, one fucking me with a huge cock while another licks my clit and another fucks me with his finger—a big finger—in my butt.

I hope I have been of some help to you. I could write lots more, but I am superhorny and would like to go masturbate.

Connie

My husband and I have just finished reading *My Secret Garden* (he did most of his reading in the bathroom; I read it usually lying on the couch). I felt I'd like to share some of my fantasies with you. But first let me tell you a little bit about myself.

I am twenty-six, have been married for nearly seven years (not always so happily, but still married). We have a four-year-old son. I work in a radio station, without pay. I have some college. I also do some writing (fiction, poetry, the like). My home life is exceedingly dull, and were it not for my fantasies, I would soon find I could do without the usual sex altogether. (Without fantasies, I find it all quite boring, sorry to say.) I'm not excessively attractive, being somewhat overweight.

Now, let me get to my fantasies. I have several, so I will try to remember all or most of them.

I think my favorite and most successful fantasy is a bondage-rape type thing. This always starts as my husband manually stimulates my clitoris, and as the excitement builds, I transport myself out of our bedroom and into a large, dimly lit chamber. Faceless, hooded, sexless people are tightening straps to my wrists and ankles. They then gag me, and I hear a door slowly creak open. I try to stretch my taut body that I might see who has entered, but I never can see the person. (I never know if it's male or female, so I'll call it "it.") But it's dressed in long, dark, flowing robes, and it approaches me slowly as it pulls a feather from a pocket in its sleeve.

This person checks the straps and gag to make certain everything is in place, then slowly proceeds to run the feather across my breasts and down my stomach to my cunt. It starts tickling me there, laughing a deep, throaty laugh all the while. The more I struggle to free myself (oh, the pleasure), the stronger it laughs. It continues this until I am all wet and creamy and quite ready to come. Then it suddenly stops, bends down, and touches the lips gently and carefully, as though it were examining me. Then it starts a soft, gentle blowing. I am still on the threshold of orgasm, but I feel a bit more relaxed, despite the wonderful agony. (Secretly, I just love the thought of being tied up and "tortured" by a feather and a mouth and a tongue.)

Suddenly, I feel teeth biting me, fingers pulling at me, tongues (more than one, it seems) licking and eating me up.

This drives me to a frenzy that is unimaginable. (Actually, it obviously isn't, is it?) While in reality I am really quite free to move, while my husband is going down on me, I thrash and flail as would a person who is tied down and being driven beyond what the senses can bear. I love it! This is truly my favorite. I know I'd like to be fucked or eaten while tied down, although I can assure you I don't wish it to happen the way it does in my fantasy. Just very sexy.

I very frequently have fantasies of women making love to women, of men making love to men. I love to watch them in my mind. These really turn me on. But none of these does quite as well as those of me and another woman. I have real lesbian tendencies, but, as yet, have only fulfilled them in my fantasies. Someday, maybe. . . .

My second favorite, though most common and enduring, fantasy involves a semipopular singer/composer/novelist/poet whom I've never met, but who has the reputation of being mad, crazy, lusty, kinky, and nearly insatiable. I fantasize about him with other women, with men, with animals, with himself, with me. With the others, he is hard, demanding, awesome, almost brutal. But with me, he is all but brutal. He is, however, still awesome. We have oral sex, anal sex, coital sex, group sex, freaky sex, kinky sex, at great heights of passion and lust. I couldn't get by a day without him. I'll put on his records and slip into a never-never land. If I'm at work or someplace and can't get hold of myself without creating a scene, I'll almost always be able to stimulate myself mentally to near orgasm just by listening to this man's music and letting him enter me in my mind, without my ever having to outwardly appear to be doing anything except my job. It's better than a coffee break.

I hope you've enjoyed reading these as much as I've enjoyed writing them down. I never discuss these with my husband, since he finds women's fantasies a threat to his virility. By the way, I never fantasize about him.

While I was reading the book, by the by, I discovered it was absolutely marvelous getting off on other women's

189

fantasies, things my own mind had absolutely never dreamed of. Thank you so very much.

Now, back to my music and my never-never lover.

Excuse me while I COME.

P.S. My husband says he never has fantasies. How does he do it?

Elaine

I have just finished reading your book—*My Secret Garden*.

It was marvelous and like nothing I have ever read before!

Thanks to your book, I now realize that I am among a good majority! I no longer feel ashamed or guilty!

I have a fantasy that brings me to an explosive and overpowering orgasm each and every time I have it.

The doorbell rings, and I answer it; as I open the door, a good-looking young man pushes his way in, grabs me, and tells me to keep quiet and cooperate. I am shocked and speechless. He smiles and pushes me down on the couch, and his body is immediately on mine—he fumbles at my clothes, and I start to struggle with him, pleading, no please, no no! He starts panting and tells me not to waste my energy because he is going to fuck me whether I like it or not. While we are struggling, he manages to get my vital parts exposed and starts sucking my breasts and rubbing his cock against me. He gets my legs open, and I feel him slip into me with one long powerful thrust! I gasp, and so does he, and as he moves in and out of me, he starts pleading with me to answer him with my movements. "Answer me, baby, please answer me," he keeps repeating—and I do! His pleading and groaning turn me on, and I start fucking with all my might, moaning—"Yes, my God, yes!!!"

It's at this time that I have a beautiful and truly explosive orgasm that I feel from head to toe! With this fantasy, I never even have to touch myself—because it's as if it were really happening!

☐ It makes me sad when I see old, old movies on television late at night and realize that for all intents and purposes, the pill and liberation seem to have killed off romance. Films today no longer present the lovers with insurmountable obstacles that keep them apart, giving us scene after scene filled with the bittersweetness of life that brings lovers together, but separates them again after only a quick, stolen kiss. Today, James Bond has barely had a gun battle with the beautiful blonde spy than they are in bed together. If sexual freedom has been an important gain for us, it must be admitted that there has also been a loss: too easy sex, sex without emotion, the very hallmark of our time, may be sex without guilt. But it is sex without romance too.

Some women try to supply from within the romance they no longer get from the films they see, the songs they sing, the books they read. Sophie writes that her fantasies are "romantic daydreams—similar to a 1940 movie." During intercourse, she does not so much try to enhance the erotic intensity of the moment as to make the time more beautiful by daydreaming of "a kaleidoscope of colors" or floating in a still stream. Killie daydreams of an "Earth Man" lover, Libby's fantasies are about "the old white-knight-take-me-away-from-this-all syndrome" . . . Phyllis writes a letter she will never send. Each woman in this chapter, in her own way, is trying to supply something she is not getting from life—or may not even really want if she did get it. Whether these daydreams are about other women, enema experiences, or even sex with children, they are truly harmless excursions of the imagination. ☐

Sophie

I recently finished reading *My Secret Garden* and believe that for many women who have been thinking there was something wrong with them because of the thoughts in their heads, that your book will provide a great service.

I, personally, however, was a little put off by the undertone of apology throughout the book—an air of justification for something that should not need to be justified, approved of, apologized for, etc.

Women have been apologizing since Eve ate the apple for the actions of their bodies and the thoughts in their heads. I would just like to see a simple statement of "this is where women are—take it or leave it" without constant reaffirmation that "it's okay to think these thoughts."

As for myself, my fantasies are sexual, involving men other than my husband, usually men I have just met and am attracted to, or to some of my husband's very good-looking friends. But for the most part, my fantasies are simply romantic daydreams—similar to a 1940 movie—the meeting or encounter, our eyes meeting, a warm embrace, and then the fade out. Also, during intercourse, I often see a kaleidoscope of colors usually within the same spectrum, such as shades of reds or shades of yellows, and sometimes I feel as though I were floating in a still stream, then into rapidly moving water, and then over a waterfall (this one is in all different shades of blue). These are more of sexual imagery, rather than fantasy, and occur during intercourse, unlike the romantic daydreams which occur at will when I'm alone, or bored. They do not excite me sexually, but they are a delightful way to pass the time.

I am thirty-one years old, married almost ten years. We have two children. I am a teacher and part-time graduate student. I would describe my relationship with my husband as fulfilling, sexually and otherwise. I have never had sex with anyone but my husband, nor do I intend to, but after reading your book, I've become very curious as to what it would be like to have sex with someone else (ergo, the sexual fantasies about other men mentioned earlier). This curiosity, however, is just that—wondering what it would be like, rather than active sexual desire.

Good luck with your next book.

Killie

I just bought a copy of your book, *My Secret Garden*, and I can't tell you how thankful I am that you wrote it. Although I always thought masturbatory fantasy was okay, I have often thought myself downright deranged because of my "daydream" type fantasy.

I am almost twenty-four years old, a college graduate, and unmarried, though still with the same lover I have had for about three and a half years. I was always a very imaginative child, and even though I was brought up in an extremely repressive environment, my fantasy life flourished. The first fantasy I can remember is imagining myself married to the star of a certain television Western, at age six or seven. I didn't know what married people actually "did," but the unknown was always there in my fantasies.

Until a year ago or so, I thought only schizophrenics had a "fantasy life"; what I now know were fantasies, I called just "thoughts." Consequently, I never thought of myself as a very sexually oriented person, although it was just about all I have thought of most of my life.

I am indeed a "watcher"—a watcher of crotches, asses, hands, beards, and hair. I try to imagine what attractive men would be like in bed, and usually comment mentally on the ones I don't fancy, even if only about how "blah" they would be. I find erotic literature very exciting. Some favorites are *Lady Chatterley's Lover*, *My Secret Life*, some of Walt Whitman's poetry, D. H. Lawrence's story

"Love Among the Haystacks," and H. E. Bates's "The Little Farm." (!) This brings me to my fantasies of the "Earth Man." I guess the best way to describe him is a hippie Oliver Mellors (gamekeeper in *Lady Chatterley*). He is strong, but not overly muscular; simple, yet not crude or ignorant. He is of rather large build and has dark hair and a thick beard. When he holds me, I feel completely enveloped (unlike my own real lover, who's about my own size). We make love in meadows of flowers and thick, lush pine woods on a forest floor of ferns. I can almost smell the damp greenness and feel the velvet moss and crunchy leaves beneath us. Sometimes I imagine we are fucking in the rain. I really like that. (Since my three psychedelic experiences—two LSD, one mescaline—these types of details have been very important in my sensual life.) My "Earth Man" lover is not dirt-dirty, but he is unwashed. The smell of unwashed armpits and especially unwashed balls and ass turns me on very much. I am not a distinct personality in these fantasies—not any sort of "Earth Mother"—but just myself. He has a full, sensuous mouth, and kissing him slowly is delicious. His hands are strong, but shapely, and I can see them caressing me. (I do like to see myself as Renoiresque, although that's not too popular these days.) We fuck with him on top, or side by side, but a great deal of the fantasy is devoted to caressing and cuddling.

Your chapter about acting out one's fantasies was interesting, as about a year ago I met my perfect "Earth Man." I walked into a college class on the first day, and there he was. I already had a vague idea of my fantasy man, but after seeing Stan, the fantasy really took hold. I was only in the class a bit over two months, but it was agony. To "act out" or not to "act out"?! I made several small gestures of interest, and thought I saw some positive response in him, but I hadn't the nerve to do anything really bold, and the class was over, and I moved away all too soon. Alas—but maybe it's better this way. I still have my dreams, which are probably better than the real person, especially when it would mean going out behind my current boyfriend's back. Still, I get a thrill when I see a guy who looks like my "Earth Man." Until reading your book, I thought this was somehow immature or faithless to my boyfriend, but I feel much better about it now.

I have a second type of fantasy, which has come into the limelight quite recently, and which I rarely use for masturbation: usually only daydreams. This is my seduction of a young boy. (That I was an only child—no brothers—may mean something here.) The boy is between fourteen and sixteen, and he is soft and lithe, yet not puny, with long flowing, wavy blond hair. He has very little body hair, and only the faint beginnings of a moustache. He is a virgin, and I have to teach him everything, even how to kiss. His lack of experience makes him shy but he is almost mad with horniness, and I bring him off with my hand first, after much foreplay. He can't get enough, and neither can I. I teach him different positions—a good one to start with is him on a chair, and me sitting astride him. I am in complete control and show him all the ways of pleasure I know; his erection keeps coming back again and again. Finally, after a wild night of insatiability, we fall asleep—he looks like a young angel, lying exhausted and sweating beside me, with his mane of fair hair in tangles and his young cock wet and limp. I feel rather old and wise (and very satisfied!).

I found myself beginning to act this one out too, when I recently was working with sixth-grade children. That's a bit young for my taste, but a few of the boys were mature enough to show a little bulge in their pants. One in particular struck my fancy, and I began to ask him to come to the classroom alone during free periods to help me with art projects. He wasn't much like my favorite fantasy-boy, but he was tempting just the same, and I really had to restrain myself. I guess women over eighteen could get sued for that kind of thing. Maybe in a more humanistic environment than the public schools, I'll get to try this one out someday. I see it somehow as an act of benevolence to give a boy a good, healthy, and loving introduction to sex. First fucks are usually pretty shitty. Besides, it turns me on.

I was surprised at your comment that few women have fantasies of seducing young boys. I thought it was rather more common. I guess one likes to think of herself as being in the mainstream.

I hope I haven't ruined these fantasies for myself by revealing them to you. I guess it's too late to worry about that now; if I have, I'm sure I'll come up with new ones.

Unless I'm really repressing them, I haven't had masochistic, lesbian, or zoophilia fantasies. There have been a couple of women I loved to look at, because they were soft and round (again, my "Renior-obsession") and just comfortable (like smelling cinnamon rolls baking). But I have no desire for any genital sex with a woman. My lover, however, is bisexual.

Again, my thanks for your book, your continuing research, and the opportunity to "sound-off"!!

Libby

I'm writing after reading your book, *My Secret Garden*. I'm twenty years old, white, middle class, and semicrazy, in a good way, I think. Anyway, I am living with a man I've known almost a year now. He's a good lover, the best I've ever had, and I'm satisfied and contented in his arms. I don't fantasize when I masturbate or when I fuck. I fantasize when my man is around the house but we're still apart.

I can get all my work and "creative outlets" out of the way during the day, so I'm ready for talk, love, etc. My loved one works hard at a white-collar job all day, and when he comes home, he's ready to read the text for the class he's taking, and/or working in the shop downstairs. He never excludes me from his activities;

in fact, he encourages my interest, but some days, I just really feel like making love. Sometimes we'll play seduction games, but usually I just read and fantasize that he rips the book from my hand and carries my body to the bedroom, that he takes off my clothes and fucks me on the kitchen floor, or that he unplugs the sewing machine and attacks my little body. What makes this one fantasy so nice is that it may happen, more than one would expect. I've been made love to in almost every room in the house (I recommend the bathroom), and when it happened, I was hoping it would. I think this is the most basic and common fantasy—the old white-knight-take-me-away-from-all-this syndrome—but I thought I'd write it down and send it along. Good luck.

Phyllis

Dearest Jennie: Even after more than a day, I'm still so thrilled by our shared experience that I just have to tell you so. Even though we were two women, still it was a sweet and wonderful love we had for that brief hour.

You are absolutely delicious, my darling, with that satin-soft glowing skin and marvelous figure. I loved smelling and tasting you all over your body, and my delight in this became almost frantic as we grew more intimate. How your tight throbbing nipples swelled as I kissed them! Never shall I forget their slightly rough texture as I nibbled at them in turn. And then when you murmured for me to slide my fingers down the cleft of your bottom. Sweet, your little hole there is so soft yet tight, so moist and musky. And it really excited you, didn't it, when I worked my fingertip up inside it? My finger felt good too, being in you there.

But of course it was your hot sweet cunt itself that drove me wild. You don't mind my calling it your cunt, do you? Although I guess some women feel that's a vulgar word, I don't think anything about you could be vulgar, and I like to think of your big hole as your cunt. And, oh, honey, how its inner flesh opened out as my fingers traced your slit. It quivered and grew very wet and hot. You did love having me caress you like that, didn't you? Of course you did, I knew by the way you wriggled and gasped.

And then when my mouth went right down on you. All that hair and soft flesh. The glorious smell of you, and the exciting taste of the moisture that seeped into my mouth. And—I suppose this is awful of me, but I couldn't help it—I loved having my nose crushed against your little bathroom place in your bottom and smelling the rich flavor of it. I wanted to just eat you up all over, gulp down all the liquid and substance of your body. I love all of you!

It's perfectly all right, dear, that you didn't do as much for me in return. I realized that you were too excited, and that it was all happening too quickly. Just your hands on me were enough, the touch of your fingers so soft and warm and loving. And you did go in my hole a little, and tickle the very top of my cunt where it feels so good. I had a wonderful come, when you did. As I felt you straining and heard your choked moans, when you hunched and ground your cunt and ass on my mouth, I knew you were climaxing hard, and my own cunt just flamed into ecstasy. Oh, sweetheart, it was all absolutely wonderful, and I'll never, never forget it.

Oh, Jennie, let me suck your cute little cunt again, and soon. Will you, dear? Please?

☐ The writer of the above letter finishes with a P.S. addressed to me:

"Dear Nancy Friday," she writes, "I never sent the enclosed letter, because the events it describes never happened, and Jennie would be horrified to learn my feelings about her. It's a fantasy letter about a fantasy experience. But I found that writing it this way made it all seem more real to me." ☐

Marilyn

I'm just about finished reading your book, *My Secret Garden*, which I find very good and honest. I'm eighteen and have an average sex life, but I can do without it for some while.

I picked up your book at an airport recently, after a visit to my sister (she's thirty-three), during which she told me that she had become a hooker. I was shocked, because I have always loved her and looked up to her. Due to the difference in our ages, she has always been practically a second mother to me.

My boyfriend, Howie, recently discovered I was reading your book, and after skimming through it, asked to borrow it. A few nights later when he came to my house, he had a friend with him who was named Dave. A girl friend of mine was there too. Howie asked Dave to read some fantasies out loud. I was awfully embarrassed, but that went away after a while. Maybe that gave me the courage to send you this fantasy, which I would like you to publish in your next book.

I have a one-and-a-half-year-old niece who I love very dearly. I sometimes sit with her when her mother is busy. I love her so much that I often think I would love to perform cunnilingus on her. She just lies there, gurgling and chuckling very happily. She loves me to touch her and play with her. What I like to imagine is the little smile of happiness she would show if I just put my face between her little legs and licked her. She is too young to think it would be anything different than just playing with her fingers and toes, and I would love to feel I was making her happy this way.

My favorite other fantasy is about a former fiancé. We balled several times, and that was the best time I ever enjoyed. Maybe it was because I felt safe. We knew each other a long time, and we were in love. Anyway, after we broke up (I still love him), I had sex with other guys, but I always imagine that the guy I'm in bed with is my ex-fiancé. Even if I'm not really in the mood for sex to begin with, just by bringing the face of my ex-fiancé to mind, imagining that he is the one who is kissing me, brings me to orgasm. Keep up the good work.

Moreen

First, may I say that your book, *My Secret Garden*, was great reading; it's about time someone published women's sexual fantasies.

My own particular fantasy started several years ago while I was hospitalized in the hospital in which I worked as a registered nurse. There were two doctors who came by on a daily basis to examine me. They were both quite arrogant and domineering in their mannerisms. As they examined me, they would have me remove my gown and have a great time poking about the most intimate parts of my body.

After they left the room, I fantasized that they were the patients, and I was the nurse in charge of them. My first order was to have them remove their clothing and put on one of those backless hospital gowns while I watched their every move. Next, I positioned them on an examination table and strapped their feet into the table's metal stirrups. In this position, I have a perfect view of their rears and penises. Since I'm wearing a short skirt with no underwear, I constantly bend over in order to expose myself to them, causing huge erections. After inserting a well-lubricated gloved index finger in their rears, I masturbate each of them until they ejaculate. By this time, they are begging me to continue; since my prime objective is to embarrass them, I decide to give each of them a good soap suds enema at the same time. After locating the longest, largest rectal tubes I could find, I slowly insert it until they again obtain an erection. As the warm soapy water is filling their rears, I masturbate each of them to the point of ejaculation. Just before they come, I quickly remove the rectal tube and release them to expel the enema. I laugh as both of them run to the bathroom, spurting semen as they go.

I should mention that part of my fantasy came true recently when I had to give our house doctor several cleansing enemas. He was the domineering type who had little or no respect for nurses. Believe me, he got the enema of his life; it's known to nurses as the HHH enema—high, hot, and a hell of a lot.

Wishing you the best of luck in your new book.

Janet

Your *Secret Garden* book is just great. My husband is a librarian and brought it home for me to read. I could hardly put it down once I started reading.

I fantasize constantly to various degrees. Every time I see a picture of Terry Thomas, or any man with a gap between his front teeth, I wonder what it would feel like to have my nipple stuck between those front teeth in loveplay.

Other than that one particular fantasy, you covered my sexual daydreams pretty well in your *Garden* book. I have never talked about my fantasies with other women, but I always just assumed that "everyone did it."

I am thirty, work as a secretary, and live separate from my husband, who is raising our two-year-old son. We have sexual relations with other people, but I have never enjoyed anyone other than my husband. However, in my fantasies, I am either watching two strangers making love, or my husband making love to some other woman.

Lucia

I read your first book and thought it was excellent. It said that you were preparing another book, so I decided to write about my fantasy.

I have fantasies about men and women, but mostly about women. I don't know why, but for some reason, the thought of being with another women turns me on. I am not a lesbian, as a matter of fact, I've been going with someone whom I love for a number of years. I've never told anyone about these fantasies. You are the first person.

My favorite one is about an Avon lady. I live in an apartment, and one day an Avon lady comes to the door. She has very big tits, with a slim body. We sit down and talk for a while about cosmetics. Then she starts to rub body lotions on my leg. Her hand moves up slowly until she reaches my cunt. I get her message and start to play with her tits. We take each other's clothes off, and she starts to eat me out. This part excites me the most, and the rest of my fantasy just consists of her eating me out until I have an orgasm.

I know I would never really do this, but if that's what turns me on, why not think about it? Your first book made me realize there was nothing to be ashamed of, and now I don't feel guilt afterward.

Thank you for listening and for understanding. I hope you can use this in your second book. I am looking forward to reading it.

Lilly

My daydreams are always the same, but each time the sexual parts get wilder. I dream I am always making it with my boyfriend's best friend. Whenever I see him, the dreams are really good, but when alone, they still satisfy me.

I dream that whenever the three of us go out anywhere, that I sit next to him. I fondle him whenever my boyfriend's not looking. Slowly I undress this guy in my mind and stare at his balls. After a while, the guy realizes that I am staring at him, and he knows what I want. Somehow we manage to get away from my boyfriend, and no matter where we are, me and this guy find a little attic. We do all kinds of neat things to each other, but there is absolutely no conversation at all, just acid music playing slowly. Once we start to really get going, I never see his face again, just big shoulders and cute belly. We satisfy each other like no other lover has ever done before, and when it's over, we get dressed, turn the music up, and just talk, like we are mere friends (even though we're not).

(End of dream.)

I dream this all the time, about the same guy, but I don't ever get upset about not being able to have him in real life. I am afraid that he won't satisfy me that much, and then my dream would be wrecked. Although sometimes I do crave his body, and I get upset.

Wilma Jean

Thank you for a terrific book. I just finished reading *My Secret Garden*. It turned me on, but I also laughed and cried. So sad that so many of us feel compelled to hide or apologize for our thoughts and sexuality.

I'm twenty-five and a mother of two. I fit into quite a few of your categories of various kinds of fantasy. I fantasize almost constantly, I've masturbated since I was twelve and really became interested in sex from about age nine. My parents never told me anything about sex and were very cool to each other. That added to my curiosity.

My husband and I really dig oral sex. I'm so surprised that many chicks I know don't like it. I daydream about performing cunnilingus on girls. The opportunity has never arisen, but I think I could dig it.

I would definitely love to make it with other guys. So many guys I see turn me on. I think about sex a lot in the daytime. Actually, I love all the aspects of sex that are pleasurable. I'll never know why people must judge each other. If they're not hurting me, I say—let them enjoy themselves!

I'm looking forward to your next book. Good luck. Thank you again.

CHAPTER SIX

MASTURBATION

☐ One of the delights in working on this book is to find evidence of the great change that has come over women in the few years since I completed research for *My Secret Garden*. Most letters I get nowadays show an absence of guilt, a sheer exuberance in sex as one of the joys of life to which every woman is entitled. It has been suggested to me that the big difference between the women in this book and the ones in *My Secret Garden* is that my most recent correspondents all read the first book. "When they saw that sexual fantasies were not just some freak idea of their own," a psychiatrist friend said to me recently, "but were in fact very widespread, and of sufficient importance to merit publication in a hardcover book—that gave women the big okay to send you their wildest ones."

I think this may be partially true, but I think the women's movement is a much more important factor in introducing a new feeling of freedom into our lives. Many women have written me that they began sharing their fantasies with their husbands long before they read *Garden*. Almost invariably, they add that they cannot see why men are put off by my work, because their husbands have always found their fantasies the hottest turn-on. If so many women and men were into sexual fantasies before *Garden* was published, it is not mere modesty that makes me disclaim the credit my psychiatrist friend wanted to give me. We are living in a new age.

It is no accident that one of the saddest letters I received is from a woman of another, older, generation than the majority of my contributors. Emma is forty-five and her letter reminds us that women have only recently begun to emerge from the centuries-old load of guilt and repression that society has laid on evil Eve and her descendants. For some women, liberation comes too late.

Emma's letter shows a combination of hope and defeat that touches my heart. It speaks of frustration and despair, of a life largely wasted for no reason except that Emma herself feels religion and society will it so. "Please do not identify where I am from," she begins her letter, fear and anxiety coming forward with her very first words. "My psychiatrist recommended your book, *My Secret Garden*, for me to read. I read it slowly to learn from it. I wish I were like the women you wrote about. I wish for better sex. I try. I am frigid, I guess. . . ."

Later in her letter, Emma goes on to give us a clue as to who might be the really frigid one in her family: "My husband and I," she writes, "have no communication. He is the boss, and to him, women are dumb and inferior to men."

I have received many letters from women telling me that, like Emma, *Garden* was recommended to them by their psychiatrists with the hope that reading it might encourage masturbation. This was suggested not only for the excitement and release of masturbation (which, along with most psychiatrists, I believe is an absolute sexual value and experience in itself) but also as a first step toward, and rehearsal for, orgasm.

While Emma may feel thwarted in her sex life because so little sexual stimulation is offered her, it is ironically true that many women today are becoming equally frustrated, because, while sex seems to be all around them, it is not the kind they will accept. Now that we are getting the idea that we women exist and can exercise judgment for ourselves, we are becoming more choosy about whom we go to bed with. The days of feeling that we have to give ourselves to anyone who asks are over. Being special, however, has its price. Special women want special men. There aren't many of them. Frustration is the result, and masturbation is most often the answer. Spending the evening at home and masturbating if the desire strikes may be a lonely form of sex, but it beats going out with any old man just because he's a man. And it certainly beats fucking him just because he's bought you dinner.

Many women have written that when they have grown bored or tired of their own sexual fantasies, they open *Garden* to find stimulation in the erotic reveries of other women. Some say that *Garden* is "nothing but a jerk-off book." I do not find this description offensive. While I hope the book is more valuable than this put-down phrase tries to make it, I am, on the other hand, pleased that it can provide such a human and necessary service. Even though Venice tells us that she was "liberally" brought up in sexual matters, she did not feel free enough to masturbate manually, even when the mood was upon her. She says it was " a mechanical thing" for her, merely letting the bathtub tap water stream onto her clitoris "sufficiently long (one-half to one hour) for release. . . ." It was only when she read *My Secret Garden* that she realized that what had been missing all along to make masturbation come alive for her "is fantasy! . . . Nothing beats imagination," her letter says. ". . . I have at last recognized the tip of the iceberg of my own fantasies."

What better way to learn about our own sexual responses than by experimenting with our desires and wishes when alone with our bodies? Many women have written me that they are unable to fantasize; it is my belief that these are exactly the people who need the most help in learning to masturbate successfully. Masturbation without fantasy is too lonely.

Little wonder so many women found *Garden* helpful. Out of our private encounters with ourselves, we learn the self-confidence necessary for the best kind of sex with someone else. "Masturbating is good for you," writes Dorothy with more native sophistication than her language shows, ". . . because if a person can make herself or himself feel that way, think how much better it will feel when another person is doing it to you."

Liberated Lady writes that she had a child and had been married for over two years, but never had a climax. While she had always enjoyed sex, she says, it was only when she decided that "it was high time I educated myself as far as what [orgasmic] response really is" that she began to understand herself sexually.

If the study of human history is all too often a record of crimes, folly, and disaster, the near universal prejudice against masturbation stands out as perhaps the one greatest producer of unnecessary suffering, anguish, and guilt. It has been proven again and again both medically and scientifically that masturbation has absolutely no harmful effects on the mind or body—unless you call feeling alive and stimulated "harmful." On the other hand, Kinsey found in his monumental researches that people who began to masturbate at an earlier age than others led more vigorous sex lives thereafter and continued their sexual activities long past the time when the average person had long since stopped having any sex at all. The evidence is clear: far from being harmful, there is a positive correlation between masturbation and sexual vitality.

One might think that given the great Female Imperative that we must remain virgin until we marry, society might have allowed women masturbation as a form of private, harmless release with absolutely no risk of unwanted pregnancy at all. Needless to say, just the opposite is true. Young girls are continually given lectures against premarital sex, but masturbation isn't even mentioned—it is a subject that is so taboo for women that mother can't even voice her prohibition.

I regret to say that we women don't help each other about this even when we are grown. I have had women friends willingly confess to me the most extraordinary sexual peccadillos—affairs and escapades that would have landed them in the newspapers, if not the morgue, if they were discovered. They have told me these stories with a quiet smile of pride, with an air of confidence that expected admiration. But only the most sexually outspoken of all my women friends have ever mentioned masturbation, and that was when I brought up the subject myself. It still remains the greatest taboo of all.

Because sexual fantasies derive much of their hidden sweetness from breaking taboos, I am not surprised by Noranna's letter about the pleasures of masturbating with a friend watching—I am more surprised that I did not receive more fantasies like hers. While she conceived of the idea and brought it to life in reality, she likes to remember it in fantasy. □

Emma

Please do not identify where I am from. My psychiatrist recommended your book, *My Secret Garden*, for me to read. I read it slowly to learn from it. I wish I were like the women you wrote about. I wish for better sex. I try. I am frigid, I guess, but desire good sex. I would welcome any of the fantasies I read about to come true in my real life (except for the whips and painful ones).

My following facts are true. I am forty-five years old (husband is too), and we have been married twenty-eight years. (Married too young because I was pregnant with his baby.) Since then we have both finished college (him years ahead of me) and have two children who have finished college and are away from home, with one still here. The only thing my husband and I have accomplished together is these three fine children. My dad is living, and I do not hate him. If something was in my childhood to make me frigid, I do not remember it. *I have never reached an orgasm with a man, or by masturbating.* I have considered the Masters-Johnson Clinic in St. Louis.

My husband and I have no communication. He is the boss, and to him, women are dumb and inferior to men.

I have considered divorce, but our religion does not approve.

I have read *The Happy Hooker, The Story of O,* etc. They are very interesting, but I do not get excited enough to reach orgasm. My husband has about given up that I ever will and is very passive (probably feels rejected, as I do, too). There is a French saying you have probably heard that goes, "There is no frigid women, only poor lovers." I would like a lover, a dog, or another woman, but where does a woman who never goes anywhere but to church, PTA, and the grocery store, etc., find this? I know of no houses with male prostitutes, and my husband would actually kill a man (and probably me) if he would learn I had been with one. So the only way would be for the man to not know my name. (We are actually prominent, successful people in this seventy thousand population town. If we moved around and didn't have such roots, I might have an opportunity.)

Both my husband and I are the same size and weight as when we married, and I feel we look a few years younger than we are. I am on birth control pills, so have no fear of an unwanted pregnancy. (But if I did have one sexual activity with a man outside of marriage, it would be sure with my luck, I would get v.d.) I am sad my sex life is not better.

As you can see, I have not excluded the idea of sex from my life even if my life is barren of sexual pleasure. I tell myself I am incapable of sexual fantasy, but even the fact that I have outlined above to you various ideas of sex with other people . . . I suppose this does mean I too have my fantasies. They are simply to feel that exquisite pleasure that must be orgasm, to feel aroused by someone or something . . . a pleasure that must be everyone's due. At this point, I would indeed gladly pay for a man's pleasure, and only wish there was such a thing as male prostitution in our culture. I am sure that once in the hands of an experienced lover I could feel all the things I have dreamed of one day knowing.

Venice

Thank you, thank you for writing *My Secret Garden*. I saw you on a television show, but when I went to buy your book, I couldn't afford the hardback price. What a mistake! Anyway, yesterday I saw it in paperback and started reading it this morning. Now it's three in the afternoon, and I *had* to stop reading. So far I have masturbated manually for the first time using just my finger (being twenty-two and brought up liberally, I thought something was wrong because I *couldn't*), called my husband home for lunch for a fine "regular" orgasm, masturbated manually in the tub, and finished with two more orgasms in my usual stream-of-water way. I had been using this for years, but it was a mechanical thing—waiting sufficiently long (one-half to one hour) for release, and what I have been missing is fantasy! I have been turned on by porn and smokers my husband brought home for us, but nothing beats imagination. I admit today I "helped" by reading your book, but I have at last recognized the tip of the iceberg of my own fantasies. Just for the record, I get off on animals and big black men (I'm white and once had a black lover). Who knows, I may find more tomorrow when I read the second half! Dr. van den Haag says on the cover that your book is of "considerable scientific interest." BULLSHIT! Science be damned! I'm interested in sex! If my cunt wasn't sore, I'd still be at it. Instead, I'm going to call my girl friend and make sure she buys a copy *today*, at any price. If praise is the word for effort, please accept mine, and yes, my love.

P.S. If this disorganized letter seems a little shaky, it's because I still am.

Libby

Today I bought a copy of *My Secret Garden*, and I've read about half of the book. I think it is fantastic—a book every woman should read!

I see myself in parts, particularly the running faucet

in the tub! That is how I masturbate too, and while reading the book, I became so aroused that I just stopped and went into the tub for some sexual release! My fantasy was that my half-brother had just come into the bathroom while I was in the tub. He was talking over his shoulder to his wife as he came in so he did not see me in there. He has already unzippered his fly and has his penis out, ready to pee. He closes the door behind him and turns around to do his business. Instead, he sees me, naked in the bathtub! I am holding my fingers to my lips, to shush him, and he quickly gets the idea. I swivel around in the tub, so that my legs are open, not to the water flowing out of the faucet, but to the stream of pee that arcs out of his cock and hits me right in the clit. (Incidentally, I have been to bed with him several times, and he's definitely *good!*)

This may not be much of a fantasy, but since no one was around, and I wanted to be balled, it really got the job done!

Thank you for making it possible to write this.

Dorothy

Hi. I'm eighteen years old and really oversexed, but it's a lot of fun. I don't remember hardly any times I've fantasized while I was fucking, but I do when I masturbate. When fucking, I just get into the guy and how it feels and the sounds; it's really nice.

I think I was three or four when I started masturbating (maybe younger), but the first time I really got off was the day I'd been to the doctor and saw a baby getting a shot, and I went home and masturbated and thought of what his little butt looked like.

Masturbating is good for you really (although some people don't agree), because if a person can make herself or himself feel that way, think how much better it will feel when another person is doing it to you.

When I masturbate, my fantasies are being fucked by

(the father of my baby) this guy I really love, or this guy I went out with a couple of years ago who was really good-looking and 6' 4", and in the fantasy, he has a really gigantic prick, the biggest I've had. (I wish I'd had a chance to really find out.)

And sometimes I fantasize that I'm a virgin (I don't think I ever was), and some guy with a really big cock deflowers me, and it hurts like hell, but I love it. The scene takes place very often in some uncomfortable place that's very small . . . like those old movies you see on television, where the bride and groom get on a train to go on their honeymoon. I imagine I just married this guy with an enormous cock, and we're in a tiny little lower berth on our wedding night. I can see that enormous powerful bulge in his pants as I begin to get undressed in there, and it frightens me. But the space is so small, how can I get away from him? By the time I'm undressed, he's taken off his pants too. I think to myself that at least I'll have a little more time, he still has his shirt on. But suddenly his cock gets even bigger, it pokes out from beneath his shirt, like a tentpole. He won't wait, and I push myself back into a corner to get away from it. But the corner just props me up all the better for him. I'm sort of sitting there, my shoulders up against the wall, my legs spread wide open in the tiny bed, and he throws himself on me. I scream as he comes at me—it's grown so big now that it looks purple and angry. In my mind, I like to make him come a little even before he's in me . . . I can "see" the little white beads of "come" spurting out, as if his cock is frothing at the mouth to get into me.

It hurts like hell. I scream, but not too loud. I don't want the conductor to hear us. He's got one hand on my mouth now so that I won't scream anymore, and the other hand is guiding this enormous piece of meat into me. He's pushing and pushing. I am afraid that my skin will tear . . . not only my "maidenhead" (in this fantasy I still have it), but even the outer skin that holds the lips together. "No, no, no," I'm half-sobbing, but nothing stops him. He's just smiling down into my face, and then with a terrific grunt, he shoves it all in, and I almost scream with the pain. It's at this point in my fantasies that I very often scream too in real life, because I've come to an orgasm.

I have this thing about big cocks. Just the way they feel being stuffed into my cunt, it really turns me on. I guess if I could have a really gigantic one, it would stop those fantasies (but I hope not).

When I was small, I masturbated with my fingers, thumb, or just rubbed my hand down there. Now I use fingers, bottle, or vibrator.

Thanks for letting me write you.

Liberated Lady

First, my background: Brought up by upper-middle-class folks . . . never participated in "sinful" activities for fear of going to hell (what a joke!). While in nursing school, I met a terrific guy from lower-middle class with no hang-up as far as participation in sex went and who had many chicks of all ages and status. Went out exclusively together for a year and a half without having intercourse (he only had two chicks in that time). My first experience with intercourse was the beginning of a new and enjoyable chapter in my life. From then on, we screwed as often as time and circumstance would permit, on the average of two times daily. Five months later, I became pregnant and after an unsuccessful attempt to abort (under doctor's care) we eloped. That was almost nine years ago. My present age is twenty-eight and my old man is thirty-one. Let's call him Z. I can truly say that I'm sexually where I'd like to be, and can attribute most of it, if not all, to Z. No one else would have put up with me for so long until I came around. I never talked about what was on my mind concerning sex or my fantasies until a year ago. Although I enjoyed sex in my own head at the time, I never had a climax until two and a half years into the marriage. What a drag as

I look back to it now. It happened almost by accident. After thoroughly reading *Of Human Sexual Response* by Masters and Johnson, I realized it was high time I educated myself, as far as what response really is. I followed diagrams of the vaginal area in detail and compared them with myself. While taking a bath one day, I let a stream of water glide over my clitoris. It felt terrific, I couldn't understand why. I stayed with it for a few moments, and bango I finally understood the damn book about climax. Shit, it blew my mind! I guess I really came to realize what frigidity was about too. For many reasons, not understandable to me, I remained cold with Z as far as my climaxing went—but completely let loose in the tub daily (and still do a lot). It only took a matter of minutes (sometimes seconds) to get off. I still have lots of hang-ups, I guess, and the faster I climax with fantasies, the better. I enjoyed watching my pelvis move almost involuntarily and my breasts and nipples get taut and pointing. I usually thought what a gas it would be for Z to be there. He'd flip. (And did when some years later he was present.) Also would imagine that the water was actually Z's tongue or a friend's hands.

Then we moved to our present home, where I got to know myself. I had everything I had once thought of as "everything"—material stuff (out-of-sight home, driver's license, and own car, pool, furniture, gardening equipment, clothes) as well as two great healthy sons and one hell of a dynamite husband. But then liberation days came around, and I too wondered what was important and why and where I was going. We got into smoking grass, and it helped me relax to a great degree. I'm a very hyperactive person. I decided to get into my head, and did with feelings and stimuli simultaneously rather than purely response. Z has always enjoyed talking about sexually stimulating things, and once I made my mind up to go with him, I found it surprisingly easy and enjoyable.

Which brings me more or less to the present. We've taken a few trips in the privacy of our home, which have also helped me to understand and accept what goes on in my head.

What did I fantasize about this morning as I was entering the climax stage? Wow! Sitting on the front porch, I had my bathrobe fully opened with the sun beaming down on my body. My hands felt cooling to my hot breasts, and as I touched my quickly responding nipples, I could feel my whole body tickle. I opened my legs wide and let the hot sun find its way to my cunt (about the same time my fingers did). I gently and slowly transferred some vaginal juices over the clitoris, which was already fattening from sheer pleasure. I sat back a bit and just watched the show. I thought of the time one of Z's friends and I were in bed together. (Just for the record, Z knew we were going to make it and encouraged it. Since then, we've had threesomes.) He had fabulous fingers and made me flip with pleasure. I continued as he did and ended up getting myself off in record time. (From start to finish: four minutes.)

An hour later, after a swim in the nude, I laid in a reclining beach chair for a smoke. The sun was still hot, and it felt great on my cooled skin. I flashed on the night before, when Z really got into eating pussy. His tongue encircled my clitoris heavenly to a climax. By this time, my fingers were taking the same path—and ended with similar results.

Then there was the time when Z and I split up for a few days, and out of the blue, the very first night alone a friend (X) came by and asked if I wanted to ball. I was taken aback, and flattered silly. It did wonders to bring my ego up to par—then some. He was eight years younger than I, and talking revealed he only made it with one other chick (his wife, who was then pregnant, X wasn't sure if it was his doings). He came on strong, embracing and soul-kissing me. His hands were all over me so quickly I couldn't keep track. It really turned me on. I had only screwed two others, but this third mate was different and very stimulating. I had thought of making it with him on a few occasions before, on a fantasy level. Because of his age, I thought it would be me who would be the aggressor, like in *The Graduate* scene. As it turned out, it was quite the opposite, and it did good things to my head, not to mention other parts of the anatomy. Every inch of me cried out for more—and more he gave. Before long we undressed, and he kissed his way from mouth to cunt in an unforgettable manner. Once he reached my clitoris, I couldn't say exactly what I thought for some time; my pelvis didn't want to stop grinding away until I was having endless climaxes. Both of us were flipping out on the experience (I didn't think I could be so relaxed and nothing but sex ran through my head for a few hours). We moved our position and proceeded to ball, which was out of sight. After a cigarette, I went down on him. It was a novelty for him that he readily got into. I found myself digging, tickling, and titillating his sensitive cock. He completely freaked over it, and wanted to stay all night. Unfortunately, we'll never make it again 'cause of circumstances as they are, but it was definitely a plus to the way I feel about sex these days.

What are my sexual fantasies? Hard to say, since most of them become reality. I dig making it with different guys, that's for sure. It opens your head up, and I can enjoy myself fuller with Z, which is where it's really at. I hold our relationship high, and all I do more or less is to strengthen and keep that relationship open and honest. We tell each other everything we do and think and fantasize.

After fantasizing about this for a while it came to a reality—I spread jelly all over my breasts and clit and let the dog lick it off. It was different to say the least.

At times, I consider myself on the frigid side, and that burns me up. Sometimes I just can't get it on, and after twenty minutes of having my cunt rubbed, sucked, and tongued, I'm on such "pins and needles" I quit the scene and go to something else. Those times are fewer now. I can remember a few times Z fell asleep after he made his deposit, and while I was lying there, his come was dribbling out of me, and it turned me on. I took my fingers and spread it all around my "pins and needles" clitoris. I thought how Z would love to see me playing like that, especially when I climaxed. Still a little bashful about that though.

Then there was the time last summer we got into vibrators. I was pushing the power mower around, cutting the grass, and thought the vibrating of the motor on the handles was perfect for clit stimulating. It was! My slacks absorbed just enough vibrations, and I climaxed.

I do think of other guys I'd like to turn on, and both Z and I have imagined ourselves with others while we are making it together. It's fun to imagine how it would really be (with friends, relatives, milkmen, etc.). They always seem to be people we know, personally, rather than movie stars or such. Maybe 'cause someday it could happen—or so I keep telling myself—who knows!

I'll go along with the findings that the most common female fantasy is submission and rape. Probably 'cause it's the only way many females will experience anyone beside their "mate." Hell, I think everyone thinks about someone different at some times. I think another reason may be just 'cause it's a onetime deal. It seems that this society looks down on screwing for the sake of screwing—and maybe they have something in that belief. Once you make it with another, the situation can get involved with their hang-ups that one just doesn't need or want. Say you ball the guy next door a few times, and that's not enough for him (or her). They make a pain in the ass of themselves—looking for more openings. Then you get to wonder about how his present mate will take it or if they can handle it. Or even if he'll tell anyone else. Hell, you don't want anyone to have any troubled thoughts over something that simply happened out of pleasure or curiosity. Swapping could be a gas, but then too you can get involved with the typical every Saturday night thing, which is a drag. Of course, this is very subjective, but that's how I feel.

I get into sex experiences of others through reading,

FORBIDDEN FLOWERS

talking, stag films, etc. I've come to realize that my
feelings and fantasies are not as rare as I thought them
to be at one time. It's comforting to know that more and
more people aren't suppressing what they actually are
feeling and thinking. I think it's much healthier that way.
I remember four years ago, when I saw my first stag film.
I was shocked! And very embarrassed, at myself mostly.
When I saw that here are females, like myself, who not
only are freer—but don't mind making movies of it. I've
felt that I'd love to be that open, but couldn't get my
thoughts into action. I don't think everyone should act
in a one, two, three manner of the "way to do things."
But, shit, that could never happen (unless they're acting).
Only if everyone accepts the way they themselves feel
are they going to make anything out of it. Too many
of us try to be someone else, and completely lose track
of where and who they really are inside.

Sure fantasies will always be there . . . thank goodness.
As to why they're there, and what to do with them, is
individually dealt with. Ask the psychologist how he
reaches a conclusion—it's usually through hearing the
fantasies of others.

I love the idea of putting myself in another's place
(maybe a hang-up again). I keep in shape and am
pleased to see myself in a mirror, tanned skin, white
breasts and bottom, and would like others to dig me too.
Sure I'd like to be in a centerfold—but that's chauvin-
istically looking at it from a feminist point of view. I
would like bigger breasts, but realize that's an old middle-
class value hang-up too. It shouldn't matter.

Hey, listen, I'm probably not making the right point—I
just can't work anymore on this. My family needs me.

Good luck on the book—hope this gets to you before
finishing it up. I'll look for it.

Noranna

I'm twenty-seven. I'm a writer, and I'm doing this
for two reasons. (1) My hubby is asleep, and I want
to get horny enough to masturbate before I join him.

218

(2) I'm egotistical enough to think my fantasies are going to be adopted by others.

Before I get into fantasies, a little background. I have masturbated since I was sixteen, and I've been with a dozen or so men. David (husband) is the best, but he's a bit of an MCP sometimes, so being really frank is proceeded slowly. Your book took us a step farther, by the way. Several years ago, a friend (female) and I admitted to each other that we indulged in masturbation, and soon we began doing it in the same room. We sort of fed on each other's sounds, which we controlled somewhat, but nonetheless could not suppress. Also, we dug on the idea that we were masturbating, but weren't alone. We always kept it darkened, but there was always enough light to allow us to see, at least in shadows, the other one with her legs spread wide open and a hand moving, caressing, rubbing a wet cunt. We especially liked the sound of the "wetness"—that squishy sound. I think women should get into this—approach the subject kiddingly if you have to, and if lesbianism hangs you up (it does me, a little), just keep in mind that you're not making love with another woman. It's just a bit of voyeurism!

Last year, I did something I slightly regret. I asked a girl I know to go to bed with me just because I wanted someone to suck on my nipples while I masturbated. I didn't do anything for her. I'm no lesbian, and she's quite unattractive, so I couldn't bring myself to reciprocate. I just HAD to have someone suck my tits hard and watch me lay there spread open so wide, rubbing my clitoris and stretching and impaling myself so deliciously on a long thick candle! She was great!

As to fantasies, I imagine that five lesbians come over and work on me. I've got one sucking and licking each tit. Two hold my legs as wide apart as they can get while the fifth eats me. This one produces a VERY large dildo. I protest that I can't take one that big, then the two holding my legs open assure me that I'll open up for it and love it that big and to relax. Number five keeps sucking my clit and just pushes it in a little. Soon I'm begging her to go all the way. Put it in me! Deep. I want it deep inside me! It's great.

I also imagine I'm at the Masters and Johnson clinic with their "fucking machine."

Sometimes my husband and I are in a film showing deprived women what they're missing, so they can get their lovers on the ball!

Sometimes I just remember my friend staring at me while I masturbated in broad daylight. It was wonderful to lay there—cunt wide open, masturbating deliciously, nipples tight and pointy while another woman watched sighing, "Wow, you don't need any help. Look at those tits! That dildo is so big. I'll bet it feels great."

Good luck on your books.

☐ Have you ever looked at yourself in the mirror and not really "seen" what you look like? You've grown so used to your features that your eyes just glide over your face without really taking note—until another person comes along and looks at you in the mirror too. Suddenly, it is as if you can see yourself with the other person's eyes. You become someone new to yourself; you examine your eyes, nose, mouth, as if seeing them for the first time. It is a strangely stimulating experience.

Some of that feeling is the emotion behind Noranna's fantasy, which is the last letter printed above. Having a friend watch her while she masturbated heightened the erotic thrill of the experience . . . made the event more real to her. Liz's and Fanny's masturbatory fantasies, which follow here, also involved observers who enhance the eroticism of what is going on. Most ". . . all of my fantasies make me an exhibitionist," Fanny writes. "When I was younger, I used to stand in front of my window naked and play with myself, fantasizing that there was a man watching me move my body around."

Many a woman's masturbatory fantasies involve a spectator, often entire audiences of people not only watching *but applauding* as she slowly and adeptly brings her to full arousal. In our usual, obvious exhibitionism—vying for attention with a new dress, a lower neckline, or higher hemline—the applause women get is for something that is *not* us: dresses or hemlines are contrived, bought, outside ourselves. Yes, the compliments we get for how we look are lovely, but how much more satisfying it would be to be complimented on our naked selves, our real selves, the erotic selves we allow ourselves to be in our masturbatory fantasies? Is it surprising that the erotic images that accompany many a woman's slow, knowing manipulation of her own body toward orgasm are those of other people viewing her at last as admirable, not because she hides her sexuality behind a pretty dress but because of her candor in revealing it to them? To be seen while masturbating can be an ultimate moment for a woman who may never have felt complete sexual pleasure, or who feels even in the throes of orgasm that her pleasure would be heightened, realer to herself, if it had not gone unseen. (Thus, the popularity of mirrors on the ceiling in bordellos.)

Even guilt, the great deterrent in reality, becomes a woman's sexual partner in a variation of these masturbatory fantasies: while bringing herself toward orgasm, she fantasizes approaching footsteps, the impending arrival of someone who will find her, catch her, "see" her. The closer she comes to being discovered, the greater the thrill of getting away with the forbidden act. The crash of orgasm, in these fantasies, comes at the very last second before the closed door is opened, the curtain pulled away, the light flicked on. . . .

A woman who signs her letter "Anonymous" gives us an unusual variation of the masturbating-while-someone-watches fantasy . . . watching her lover masturbate. This is another idea that our culture finds difficult to accept: men themselves don't think the sight of their sexuality in all its forms is exciting for women to look at.

I believe just the opposite is true. Women not only love to look at men, but they also enjoy watching them masturbate. To carry this idea to its ultimate, I also believe there are women who would enjoy watching their lovers make love to another man (as several letters in this book testify). I have found this idea difficult to discuss even with therapists and psychiatrists, but it stays in my mind with a certain symmetrical logic: men have always enjoyed watching women naked, women playing with themselves; above all, the sight of two women making love to each other is notoriously the ultimate turn-on for most men. Why then is it so difficult to reverse the roles and recognize that women would find just as much arousal in seeing two men in a circus? □

Fanny

I'm not even through reading your book on woman's sexual fantasies, but I just had to write to you and tell you that it is absolutely *fantastic*!

I never knew that there were so many woman who had sexual fantasies. I've always had them as far back as I can remember. I always felt that I was weird or oversexed.

I'm sort of caught between two generations. I'm twenty-three years old, this is my second marriage; the first time, I was sixteen and pregnant. The second time, I was nineteen and pregnant (the second time, I didn't know I was pregnant). As you can see, even though I was brought up that sex was a no-no, and you wait until you were married, I didn't. When I was fourteen years old, I was raped. Not violently. I knew both of the guys, and one of them I had gone out with for a month or so. I had never let him fuck me, but he had eaten me, and I had eaten him. (He was eighteen, by the way.) One night, I was at a barn dance in Vermont. I guess he was really mad at me, because he thought I had done it with someone else. So he and his friend got me when I went outside to go to the bathroom. I was scared at first, but he kept on saying, "wow, feel this cunt, isn't this the best cunt you've ever felt?" This was before they were inside of me, he was using his fingers and hand. That is where I started getting turned on. Then when he started fucking me, I was lost in sexual pleasure. He kept on talking all the time, saying "wow, you have a really beautiful cunt; I want to take my prick out of you and suck it, but I can't, it's too good." By this time, I was starting to scream with pleasure, and he told his friend to keep his hands over my mouth as there were other people all around us. When he was done, it was his friend's turn, and believe me, he was just as good. All the time, they were fucking me, they were talking about my tits and cunt, which made me unafraid and enjoy it. Every day I thank him for making my first time so wonderful. I guess that couldn't be called a fantasy, as it actually happened, but I often think about it, and then I masturbate. I also think that that is why most all of my fantasies make me an exhibitionist. When I was younger, I used to stand in front of my window naked and play with myself, fantasizing that there was a man watching me move my body around, play with my nipples, stick my fingers in and out of my cunt, and whack myself off right there before him, and after I finished, he would come into the house and fuck me. That was when I climaxed.

One of my fantasies now is that I'm on stage in front of a room filled with men and only about a dozen women. I come out and strip to the music; then I walk back 'n' forth playing with my tits (I usually do this in front of my mirrors to get the effect), bending over, spreading my ass apart so that they can see my two holes. By now, the men are screaming, "Come on, baby," and the women are in shock. Then I bend over backward and do the same thing, so they can get a good look at my cunt this time. Then my hands start going all over my body as my body moves to the music. Now I notice that some of the men have their pricks out and taking the situation in hand and screaming, "Come on, baby, let me see that big cunt of yours again." Now I lie down on two stools and start whacking my cunt off, making sure my legs are spread wide, so they can see my cunt jiggle, and now some of the men have dragged the women up on stage and are fucking them while they are watching me and seeing my cunt move, which makes them fuck the cunt they have all the harder, until finally everyone has made it.

Another fantasy while I'm masturbating is simply that while I'm doing it to myself my girl friend has walked in on me and joins me; then we make love to one another. This fantasy gets me very excited, but it will soon no longer be a fantasy, because I really want this girl friend. She has big beautiful tits that I would love to suck and the same with her cunt and ass. Anyway, I'd love to have this girl, and I know that she's starting to want me. We almost did it yesterday, but we didn't, because we're both on the rag. I've had sexual relations with five other women. One of them was a prostitute.

One thing I want to say before I close. My husband knows of my fantasies and approves and gets very excited over them. Sometimes we lay in bed, and while I play with myself and he plays with himself, we tell each other some fantasy and come together. He also approves of me going to bed with a broad and sometimes watches us, and I watch him play with his big prick, then afterward we fuck; if the girl has her boyfriend there, they fuck too; if not, we wait till she leaves or we leave, depending on the circumstances.

I hope that I have been helpful toward your second book. Thank you for letting me contribute.

Liz

For years, I was resentful that man thought he could write about women's sex life as if what he wrote was fact. You're right up top . . . for the first time, an honest woman putting the real facts on paper. When I read your book, I said, "Now that's the truth." Only a woman knows the sexual fantasies of other women.

Here's my favorite. My lovers in this fantasy are faceless, and I have dreams where I am sitting with black mesh hose on, the kind that have black heels. I'm on a tall chair, no bra, and I caress my round firm breasts and pull and pinch my erect nipples. I feel extreme pleasure in my womb to do this, and then I spread my legs, and the slit in my stockings shows love juices oozing out of my pussy's lips. They are large and hanging down like a pink tongue panting to be fucked. A naked man is there watching me play with myself, but I do not see him; he is silently watching me until I am dying to be screwed. He gets a fantastic erection watching me. I just want to be yanked off my perch and screwed so hard on the floor that I'm dying with pain and pleasure. I can feel it so clearly, his beautiful hairy mound bumping against my love venus. He is moaning and blowing his hot breath in my ears, and the heat is so intense when he comes, and I feel the hot juice shoot up around my cervix. It leaps with joy, and I come, and my womb pulls and sucks his juices up in me like a thirsty throat on fire. I feel my cunt, and it's running down my legs—I rub it and it's tender. I'm always hot and masturbate often with this fantasy, even though my husband is fantastic, with a beautiful peter.

He drew me out of my shell and nurtured my sexual freedom—I can say I've had other men in real life, but my husband excites me by far the most. I love him and he loves me. The fact that he has other women runs my cunt pressure to the boiling point, and I desire his hot big beautiful peter even more, as I fantasize he is screwing *her,* and when he says, "Fuck me, baby," or "Suck that hard hot cock, baby," I know he's talking to her. But I know I'm better in bed than she is, and my excitement transmits to him, so it's an electric charge shooting back and forth. It's a current that I drink—my life's blood. I love all of him.

I discovered my sex drive while very young, because I lived on a farm and watched the animals mate. I never desired any of these myself, and yet the reptile played a most delightful wicked part of my fantasies. This one takes place when I was twelve or fourteen years old. I'm lying in bed on fire with an itch that drives me crazy. In my fantasy, I think, What can I fuck and my parents not know, even though it is right under their nose (my mother was a very light sleeper)? I have it—a snake.

It slithers quietly and surely on its way. I'm lying on the bed, naked, hot and wet, all swollen with yearning. It slides under the door, long, big, and hard and wicked—(the devil!)—creeps on the bed without effort and drives its ugly head right into my throbbing hot pussy. The thrill knows no end as I masturbate faster to keep in time with the shivering snake.

I had this fantasy for years till I got married. Then it switched to men and real penis dreams.

P.S. These are only a few. I could go on. As some of the other women in your book said it gives me great pleasure to read and write some of my most secret thoughts. Your title is most appropriate, as I used to fantasize I was floating through a lovely flower garden while my husband screwed away. Such a lovely flower garden.

P.P.S. As for facts, I married at seventeen. I was a virgin, have two sons now, and am thirty-eight years old. If I had to have a removal of my female parts, it would surely make me die. I believe the womb plays the most important part in having a climax. As the Greeks said, when you translate "womb," it means a living thing—thirst.

Anonymous

Just finished your book and couldn't resist sending you my favorite fantasy. Although it's based on fact, I conjure it up when I'm alone and getting it on by myself or with my friendly little vibrator. I'm married but have had a lover for a very long time. I love my husband but I have this leftover sexual desire that he—and maybe no one man—could ever satisfy. I don't dig cheating on him, but it's better than frustration. My lover and his wife, my husband and I, and several other people we know all form a kind of close-knit group, and so we very often do lots of things together. Many of us like to ski, and last year, one of the couples in our group invited my husband and I, and my lover and his wife, to come north for a weekend of skiing with them.

They have a small weekend house, with a combination living room and kitchen, one large bedroom with two double beds side by side and two single beds. At first, I thought, Shit—there is nowhere in this little house where my lover and I could hope to get anything on.

We skied all day and were totally exhausted but feeling sexier than ever. We had tried to get off on the slopes alone, but someone was always tagging along with us. It was a great night. A big fire in the fireplace, drinks, soft music, and me—ready to screw anything that moved. I had almost resigned myself to making it with my husband, which wouldn't have done me too much good, but I was desperate. We all went to bed. My husband took some sleeping pills (he has insomnia). So there I lay in one double bed and my lover fifteen inches away in the other double bed. I was going crazy.

Could I kneel on the floor and go down on him without anybody hearing or seeing us? No, that's out. Just then, he must have been reading my mind. He pulled back the covers and turned on his side, and there was the most beautiful hard-on in the world. I was going to get down on the floor and the hell with anyone else. He motioned for me to stay where I was and then started to jack himself off. Right then and there I knew what he had in mind. I turned over on my side as close to the edge of the bed as I could. My heart and everything else was beating like a trip hammer. I was so wet and my clit was so hard, I thought it would burst. Then he started to come and cupped his both hands to catch it all. He then brought his hands up to my mouth, and I proceeded to lick them bone dry, not wasting a single drop of that lovely stuff. Between picturing in my mind him jacking off and that warm, slightly salty semen in my mouth, and of course the danger in what we were doing, I got off twice. I drifted off to sleep with his finger in my mouth.

Now when I masturbate, I think of that scene, and it's almost like having him there. Given a good husband, a good lover, *and* my fantasies, I'm never frustrated. I hope you can use this. It would be an even bigger turn-on reading about it. Plus knowing all my friends were reading it and not even knowing it is about us. Thanks for bringing fantasy out of the closet, and crotch-watching too.

☐ Have you ever listened to an older person talk about "the good old days"? To hear them, the men were all tall, kind, and rich, the women beautiful and generous as queens, the rain never fell on weekends, and every night was New Year's Eve. To say that they are telling us lies would be incorrect and narrow-minded. What they are trying to do is recapture a feeling they had when they were young, and which they have no more. They are not deliberately misleading us as much as they have embellished their own memories of a world that should have been. They themselves can't be sure if a certain happy event, which they describe in such glowing detail, really happened or not.

The next two fantasies may be based on just such memories. To be honest, it is not clear to me if Diane's or Cecelia's fantasies are about events that really took place, or if both women have not taken some specifics out of real events and, because they ignited such truly erotic fires in their imagination, embroidered them into two of the most vivid masturbatory fantasies I have ever read.

For our purposes, it does not matter, because whether or not the events took place, both fantasies are true to their own inner logic. Diane does not even present her story as if it were a fantasy. It is all memory, and whether it is about masturbation, dogs, her grandfather, another woman, a casual newsboy, or a salesman, the details all pour out, one after another, with no hesitation, second thoughts, or guilt getting between herself and her mounting excitement. The very act of writing the letter becomes part of her total masturbatory fantasy: "Our dog gets his share, and he can lick my cunt as he is doing right now, while I am writing."

Cecelia's story seems to me to be a bit more complicated. I have shown it to two psychoanalysts, both of whom share my feelings that it is difficult to know just by reading her letter where reality ends and fantasy begins. If the events actually happened, it can be said that she was legally and technically "raped," but I believe it would be a total misunderstanding to believe Cecelia is the exception to my statement that I never met a woman who wanted to be raped in reality. In her letter, she tells us where her true excitement lies: it was "the enslavement, the subjugation—[which] I found so thrilling." When she wants to experience these emotions again, she does not go out alone for a walk on a dark street—she turns to "the understanding and indulgence of my wonderful husband" to turn her fantasy into "a way of life," in the safety of her own home.

What is particularly striking to me about Cecelia's letter is that it gives us such a clear example of the healing powers of sexual fantasy. By going over and over again "eleven hours" of "terrifying brutality," Cecelia gets a feeling of mastery over the events. She can resummon those hours in her imagination now for her own pleasure. Her erotic imagination has taken the horror out of her experience, and transmuted it into pure sexual gold. She says the entire experience now "thrills me to think of." In the safety of her fantasies, the man who abducted her can no longer frighten her; they have been turned instead into her erotic servants, Cecelia's source of "extremely satisfying pleasures." □

Diane

Your book, *Secret Garden,* is very well fitted for its purpose. My gramps and I have read and reread many parts and many of the fantasies fit my life. Am twenty-three, single, and have had a varied sex life. My remembrance of sex-play must be when I was about six years old. Every chance I had when alone was to strip all my clothes off, sit with my legs up to my chin, and just finger play. At the time, the words cunt, fuck, cock, etc., were not my language, but now I know and shall use the proper word in my letter. The sex-play I enjoyed was to use my finger, and then I tried many items, rubber items for pets, such as is given to dogs to chew on. Well do I remember finding a big rubber cock in a box in the storage room. I kept it well hid and played with it after I had gone to bed. The size was large, but in a short period of time, I had mastered getting it way up in my cunt. The time I had it up my cunt when our dog came into my room, jumped up on the bed, and—as your book described—a fast lick with a doggie's tongue, and your new experience is in for a thrill. Well, after that, whenever I could be alone, I would let Skip lick my cunt. Could be in our garage, basement, or in the woods, as we lived in the sticks. He was always ready to lick my cunt. From that, I soon learned he loved to hug my leg and work his ass. Well, I had him on his back one day and played with his cock. No one home, so I stripped and sat on his stomach and slid my cunt up to his cock and let it go in. It was real warm. I worked my cunt on his cock, and he laid still. His head was behind me, so I could hold him and force his cock in. While I was only eight then, I had seen dogs fucking, so I was anxious to see if he could fuck me. We went for a walk back into the woods and found a spot where we would be not so apt to be found. Now I never wore panties, and all I had on was a dress. I took off my dress and spread my legs apart while standing, and let Skip lick my cunt. When he got to working his ass, I got down on my knees to get him to fuck me. He knew what I was doing and mounted me. I got my hand on his cock and spread my cunt open and led his tip of his cock into my cunt. What a thrust he gave, and my cunt was full of his cock. Every stroke he gave, his cock got longer, and then I felt a bulge go in my cunt, and we were in action. Sure glad no one was around to hear me talk like I did. When he got going, I kept telling him to fuck faster, faster, faster, and it seemed so much pleasure. Finally, he came, and when I started to pull away, he cried; I could feel the hardness just inside my cunt. When he pulled his cock out of me, my cunt was on fire, and was his cock slender, but long. The huge knot at the back end of his cock was bright red. I laid on my back and just let my cunt cool, as it was really hurting. He licked my cunt, and when he found my clit, he just kept licking. Guess my juice was coming, and he was licking it as it came out. Well, we have had many a good fuck since, and I found another dog to replace Skip. Well, when I was about eleven years old, our newsboy came to our house to collect, and everyone was gone to Seattle. He and I talked for a while—he was sixteen then—and while he was talking, he gave me a hug and kiss, and left. Shortly after, he returned and explained he had to finish his collections. We were in my room playing records, etc., and he started to fool around, and that was all I needed to get my cunt hot. In our playing on the bed, he got his hand on my cunt, and that was where I lost all respect. I stripped and let him do what he wanted. My tits were small, but he found a way to suck both. Then he had me lay crossways on my bed, put two pillows under my ass, and had my cunt up high. I could see my cunt lips open up when he spread my legs. When he put his mouth to my cunt and started to suck my clit, I grabbed his head and pulled his head up to my cunt, and as he sucked, I kept telling him, "Suck, suck harder." Finally, he came up on top of me and told me he was going to fuck me, and he got his cock up in my cunt, and when he started to fuck, my legs were over his shoulders, and did we fuck. This was our start to fucking. Did he get a look of surprise when Skip came up and licked his cock and nuts while he and I were fucking later on. Skip, Ted, and I are now a threesome for a long time after. When Ted was eighteen, he joined the service and is now making a career of the Air Force.

Well, by then, I was thirteen years old and as hot a bitch as could be found. Ted told me to be careful who I fucked, as I could get a disease. When Ted left for training, I was without a fucking partner. One day, I had fantasies about my grandpa and that he fucked me. He lives about ten miles from our house, but visits us often, so I decided to ask Gramps about coming to his house for a day. That worked out, same day I left my panties off after I got to his house (he lives alone), and he soon found out, because I made it a point to let him get a look at my cunt. That afternoon, he told me he was going to give me a bath, as I was needing one. He did, and our sex life began. He sure enjoyed my body, and my tits were becoming big. Well, now it has been ten years, and Gramps and I still have our sex. He taught me cleanliness, hygiene, and care of my period, keeps my cunt shaved, and loves to fuck. He and I go down on each other; he taught me to suck cock. And when he gets a notion he gets a new sex toy, dildo, vibrators, double-end cocks, so my girl friend and I can stick it into our cunts and play around. Gramps found her when he was at dinner, and she loves to stay as a lesbian. When Gramps comes to our house (Sue and I live together), we sure give him pleasure. He fucks one of us and sucks the other cunt. He has always given both of us the best in fucking, sucking, finger-fucking, vibrator, or, may we say, just a lot of sex fun.

Forgot to mention I am a dress designer and do a great deal in designing exotic gowns. Some I design are about as bold as can be to expose titties, ass, and some are designed to expose the cunt. When I do fitting, I have the lady stripped, so I can hold the breasts for measurements or to fit around cunt. Several times I have excited them to a point where they want me to play with the tits and cunt. A few have asked me to strip, and they have gone down on my cunt. Guess my shaved cunt must excite them. Yes, I have sucked a few cunts and tits. Gramps and I are enjoying our sex life. He did not have to ask me to suck his cock, while showering together, I just could not resist taking his cock and sucking it. He invited both of us to go to see *Deep Throat*, and after we got home, we bet Gramps one of us would be able to take every inch of his huge cock and swallow the head. Well, we surprised him by being able to do just that. Fantasy has never entered my mind. I suppose you could say I live my fantasies as they come into my head.

Gramps has fucked us both in the asshole. My roommate had a cousin visit us from San Diego, and what a wild fifteen-year-old she was. She had a cunt on her one-hundred-eight-pound body that we shaved and gave her a suck off, and she responded by doing our cunts the same. So, Nancy, guess in my sixteen years, I have had as much of a variety of sex, never wear panties, and love to spread my legs so the guys can get the bulge of a hard cock and then leave.

Now use my letter or throw it out, but I know now that women are not only willing to tell their story about the sex they enjoy, but love to read of other cunt action.

When Gramps and both of us are in bed we never feel a bit bashful to suck a cunt while being watched.

Our dog gets his share and he can lick my cunt as he is doing right now while I am writing. After I get fucked, I love to spread my legs in the shower. I piss a stream anywhere it goes. Gramps sits down in front of me when I piss standing and I piss all over him, and he sucks me dry.

Enough said.

Cecilia

I can't tell you just how comforting and reassuring it was for me to read your book. I had for the past three years harbored a secret guilt, because I found so much pleasure in reliving in my fantasies the extremely satisfying pleasure I experienced when I was abducted in a shopping center parking lot by three men, taken to an extremely secluded house in the suburbs, and raped. It was more than just rape, really. It was sexual enslavement for about eleven hours, and it is that—the enslavement, the subjugation—I found so thrilling then and which I not only fantasize now but, thanks to the understanding and indulgence of my wonderful husband, have turned into a way of life. Perhaps you can understand the sense of guilt I have been suppressing—until I read *My Secret Garden*—because I enjoy his domination over me and my regard for him as "my lord and master." (My girl friends, most of them more into women's liberation than I ever could be, laugh when I use that phrase and feel I'm making a little joke when I use it, but I'm much more sincere about it than they could ever realize.)

First of all, let me say that I had been rather inhibited in my sex life prior to that night I was abducted, but I wasn't a virgin. My fantasies, even then, centered around the slave-girl theme. I have always read novels and seen movies in which the beautiful heroine is bought at a slave auction by the handsome Roman commander or the ancient Egyptian prince or something like that, but always kept them more or less in check when I fantasized myself in the situation (although I did use them when I masturbated). But that night opened a whole new world for me sexually, and eliminated virtually every inhibition you can dream of.

Parts of that night still remain a blur to me. I was so frightened for a large part of it, especially the early part when I didn't know exactly what was happening and was beaten—though not too hard—until I agreed to submit and be obedient—and toward the end, when I wasn't certain that they would ever let me go. But in between, I slipped into my fantasy and actually became that slave girl I had fantasized about. I lived the role. It was as though I had been transported back across the ages to ancient Rome or from reality into a novel or movie.

It is this that I recall vividly now in incredible detail, four or five of the things that happened to me especially which thrill me just to think of them now and which I fantasize about constantly and which my husband duplicates as well as possible, but without the terrifying brutality of that night.

I was twenty-three and single. I had my own apartment and was working as a receptionist in a law office and was doing some fashion modeling part time in the evenings when I could. They took me as I was getting back into my car after buying groceries at a supermarket. They just shoved me into my car onto the floor in the rear and drove off with me. There were three of them. One was about twenty-five or twenty-six, and was the leader or, at least, the one who told the other two what to do and who gave most of the orders to me. He was very soft-spoken and suave, but extremely firm and commanding. The other two were still in their teens, I suppose. One was a huge guy, dark and hairy and very strong. The other was very good-looking, blond, and had very smooth skin.

They drove into a garage and pulled me from the car into the house. I don't remember too much of what happened—I was just so terrified, but they stopped hitting me, and I agreed to do whatever they wanted and had slipped into my slave-girl fantasy role, these are things I remember with incredible detail and which I fantasize about still.

1: I was still fully clothed, and I was made to stand in front of the two younger ones as the older one walked about me, touching my hair lightly, my face, my breasts, my throat. He kept talking, telling me how pretty I was and how much he was going to enjoy fucking me. He began unbuttoning my blouse and finally slipped it over my shoulders, commenting on how beautiful my skin was and how nice my tits were. He ran his finger lightly over my shoulders and circled my breasts and finally touched the tip of my nipples. He brushed them with the knuckles of his hand and took them between his finger and thumb and rolled them very gently, embarrassing me by telling the other two that my nipples were becoming erect. It was such a pleasant sensation I couldn't avoid squirming, and he commanded me to be still. I began crying quietly. I remember distinctly when he put his hand under my skirt and began stroking the insides of my thighs. His voice sounded so dirty when he told the other two that I was "creaming through my panties." But, oddly, I loved the sense of humiliation. He finally made me take off my skirt and my panties "very slowly, so we can watch your tits as you bend over." Then I had to stand naked in front of them and turn slowly, so they could look at me. And I knew exactly how that heroine slave girl in my fantasies felt as she was being auctioned.

2: I was lying on the floor and the big one was lying across me, perpendicular to my body. He was toying with one nipple with his hand and licking the other. The older one told the young blond one to lick my cunt. The older one lay down next to me and began kissing my face and stroking my hair. All the sensations were driving me out of my mind. I have never before—or since—had so many fantastic things happening to my body at one time. I couldn't concentrate on one. I tried to ignore them, but I couldn't. I'd try to think of something else—how much I hated these men—but then the blond one would suck on my clit and flick it with the tip of his tongue, and I would just feel him and what he was doing, and then the big one would circle my nipple with his tongue, and then the blond one would move his tongue very rapidly back and forth across my clit. They kept saying things like, "You like to have your clit sucked, don't you?" and "You like having your tits and your cunt licked at the same time, don't you?" I'd try to ignore them, but there was no way in the world you can ignore the moist warmth of a soft mouth gently, persistently exciting your clitoris. I tried desperately to suppress having an orgasm, but the older one kept encouraging me. "Go ahead, baby, come, baby, come. You love it." And I came. It was so deep and intense. It was fantastic. (I get hot just thinking about it and writing this letter. I'm wearing ben-wa balls—those gold little Japanese balls you put inside your cunt and which vibrate when they click together and I've been unable to keep my hips still while I'm typing this and have had an orgasm while I'm typing. It's great.)

3: They took turns fucking me after that. I was still exhausted from being licked into having an orgasm and was in almost a dream, but I remember so many of the sensations. Each one of them was different and felt differently inside of me and on top of me and fucked differently. I know I came again several times. I can't remember how many times each of them fucked me or with which ones I had orgasms. The older one fucked me first, I remember. He put his prick deep into my cunt so that he was pressing very hard against my clit. He barely moved. I remember pressing my cheek against his shoulder and feeling the hardness of his prick inside me, filling me. When I moved my hips, he commanded me to "just lie still. Just lie there and feel my prick in your cunt. Just lie there and get fucked." I remember feeling an orgasm welling up inside me in spite of everything I did. I actually wound up asking him to please, please, fuck me, please let me come. I know that eventually I was thrusting as hard against him, trying to fuck him, as he was me. I actually was fucking the man who was raping me and enjoying it tremendously. The young one fucked me very rapidly, I remember, and I remember putting my legs around him, he was so slender. The big one fucked me more than once, I know. I just remember staring into his chest. It was a curiosity to me, then, just how differently each one felt and how each moved. That, in itself, I find exciting. (I had slept with only two other men before that. I was a virgin until my junior year in college, when I was twenty. I didn't like or dislike that experience. I was too curious then, I suppose. I slept with one other man three times after that. I had hoped that we would be married, but we broke up. I had dated the man I later married twice before being abducted, but we had never gone to bed together.)

4: We all rested for a while, and then the older one said he wanted to watch me sucking the blond one's prick. I had never sucked off a man before and was frightened. He threatened to cut off my tits and flashed a knife, and I finally agreed. But the blond boy either was reluctant or was pretending to be. The older one put the tip of the knife at my throat and said he would give me fifteen minutes "to have that kid come in my mouth." The boy was sitting on a sofa, and I went to him thoroughly terrified. I got on my knees, but he pushed me away. The older one said, "Coax him. Make him want it." And I found myself sitting next to him, playing with his cock, and kissing him, trying to brush my nipples against his lips to make him hot and whispering into his ear and begging him to let me please suck his prick. I was encouraging him to put his hand between my legs and was spreading my legs to make it convenient for him and telling him how wonderful I would make it feel if he would let me suck his prick. In the background, the older one kept saying, "Ten minutes left. . . ." Finally, the boy consented, and I got on my knees between his legs. I remember how hard and firm his prick was and how the smooth skin seemed to slide over the hardness of his shaft. When the older one said, "Five minutes, baby," I was sucking and licking desperately, frantically. One of them—I don't know which one—pulled my hair away from my face so that the older one could watch "his prick going in and out of my mouth better." I had never sucked a man before, but the thing I remember most about my feelings at that particular moment was that I couldn't remember ever feeling as female as then. I was thoroughly aware of the ultimate symbol of masculinity directly in front of my face, in my mouth. I was aware of the power and strength of these men over me. It wasn't just my femininity I was aware of, it was my femaleness—if that can be clear. I enjoyed sucking his prick immensely, and I enjoy being made to suck my husband's. When the boy came, I felt a sense of mastery in being a woman. I felt complete. I enjoyed it so much.

They kept me for several hours after all this. I had to wait on them, serving them pizza—they actually sent out for one, and one of them held me in a basement family room when the delivery boy arrived, with a knife at my throat (they suggested giving me to the delivery boy as a tip)—and I had to kneel after serving them wine while one of them poured wine into my mouth. I was ordered to fuck them as they lay on their backs. I don't think I came again, I was exhausted, I guess. And I became frightened as time passed, and there was no move to let me go. Finally, they allowed me to dress, and they drove me to about a block from my apartment and let me out. They parked my car back in the supermarket parking lot, and I got it the next day. I went home and bathed and slept straight through for eighteen hours after I got home. I never called the police about it.

I stayed home for three days after that and masturbated when I recalled my favorite parts of the incident, reliving them. I had a date with Larry the Saturday night after that. We were supposed to go to dinner and to the theater, but when he arrived, I told him that I wanted to stay there, and I wanted him to make me fuck him. I told him the whole story of the abduction, about how I enjoyed it. He sat in a chair and told me to stand in front of him. Then he told me to take my dress off. And that began our relationship, really. We were married a year later. When we are alone, we still play out the master-slave relationship. He'll call me from the office before he comes home and order me to undress and wait to be fucked. It is extremely pleasurable to greet my husband at the door when I'm either naked or wearing a sheer chiton and wait upon him and do loving things to him. And for him. He has a friend who stays with us over weekends several times a year while in town on business trips, and Larry always has me wear a rather seductive, low-cut cocktail dress when Frank visits. He has me light Frank's cigarettes, and I enjoy watching Frank's face as he looks down the front of my dress (Larry has forbidden me to wear bras). It turns me on also when Larry tells Frank how great I am in bed or how well I suck his prick. It embarrasses me, but it is fun. Larry also has threatened to order me to sleep with Frank during one of his visits, but so far, he has not. I will if he tells me to.

I know this may sound as though I'm pretty kinky. But for the first time in my life, I'm feeling free sexually and thoroughly satisfied. I don't have many of the hang-ups my girl friends seem to have. I'm involved in the Junior Women's Club and work as a volunteer once a week at the children's ward of the local hospital. I do all the things my girl friends do. So, can it be all so bad to find so much pleasure sexually in the way that my husband and I find satisfying? Certainly, your book would indicate that other women would love to live out their fantasies the way I do mine. They should. It feels so good. Can it honestly be so wrong? I don't think so.

Love and sincere thanks again.

Carole

I've just finished reading *My Secret Garden* and was thoroughly fascinated. I consider it the best turn-on of my vast collection of literature.

Just to acquaint you with myself, I am a single, twenty-three-year-old stewardess. And layovers are a great time for masturbating and fantasizing or fucking if you're lucky enough to know a man in that town.

I consider myself completely uninhibited and like my men that way. I sew, crochet, cook, write poetry, and read a lot. Of course, all this is between flying and fucking. One of my favorite things to do is to get a group of people talking about sex—you find out so much about them, without their knowing it.

There were a lot of women in your first book who had some of my qualities in sex (crotch-watching, good music, voyeurism, male nudes, etc.), but I didn't really find any fantasies like mine.

I don't know if it's unique or not, but all my fantasies are done in twelves. They are never involved with faceless lovers; instead, they are always past or present lovers. The twelves are sometimes mirrors in a fun house, scenes in other countries, or twelve positions. One time, it was my four best lovers in my favorite of their positions as stick people, cartoon characters, and then real-life figures (three times four is twelve).

My favorite fantasy of all has to do with the twelve signs of the zodiac. I usually have this fantasy after I've been smoking grass and during oral, manual, or vibrator sex. I always like to hear Barry White's albums in the background—I can have an orgasm just from his voice, without ever being touched.

Anyway, the fantasy starts out in Aquarius. My cunt is on fire, and the water-bearer puts it out by sticking his hose into me. As Pisces, I'm the Star-Kist tuna mermaid, and my lover is a scuba diver. Being that a mermaid has no pussy, I eagerly go down on him. As Aries, my man is a Los Angeles Ram, and I'm the head cheerleader (as what Dr. Chartham calls a practitioner of *erelalia* [noisy lovemaking] the part fits me). And we never fail to score a touchdown. Taurus brings us to Spain, where the toreador kills the bull and fucks me with its horn. In Gemini (my sign), I am being fucked by one twin while I devour the other twin with my mouth. Cancer takes us to the circus freak show, where my lover has six arms and thirty fingers. He literally pinches me to an outstanding climax. Leo, the lion, sits on his throne, and, lifting all my petticoats, I sit down on his prick. As I laugh at the jester, my vagina laughs too, and the king gets a royal orgasm. Virgo's scene is in Egypt, where I am the virgin bride in the sultan's harem. I belly dance for him, feed him grapes, fan him, and then he gently deflowers me. Libra is the scales, and two people fucking on one are never going to get the correct weight. Scorpio can be very sadistic. So, here my lover ties me to the bed, whips me, and has me gang-banged by his motorcycle club. Sagittarius, the archer, is an Indian chief who fucks me with his arrow as we ride double on his palamino. Capricorn is a shepherd in his pasture, and I become the black sheep he fucks anally.

That seems like it's long, but it takes longer to read than to think.

Well, off to Detroit and my super Gemini lover. Mmmmm. . . . Love and piece.

Gabbie

I just finished your book, *My Secret Garden*. Really fantastic. I thought it might be exciting to put my fantasy down on paper. Maybe you won't use it, but I'll do it anyway. By the way, I have had only one lover and have been going with him for four years. I am eighteen years old.

Well, I wake up in this large rather dimly lit room, and there is incense burning somewhere off. I'm sitting on some sort of apparatus attached to the walls, with my arms and legs suspended. I'm wearing a kind of harem outfit, except the bra is nothing but thin chains holding up my breasts (36C). The pants are very thin filmy material (see-through), but my bush is covered by thick bands of lace that go around the crotch.

A door opens, and this very handsome dark-haired boy comes into the room, wearing only some sort of decorative gold shield over his genitals suspended by gold chains. I ask him what I'm doing here, and he replies that his father kidnapped me so that his only son could have an American wife and child.

I was married to him earlier while hypnotized, he tells me, and had been given a drug that would make me conceive the first time the marriage was consummated. He also told me that I couldn't resist, because the incense had an aphrodisiac drug in it.

He comes toward me, and I find that I can't resist this sexily bodied man of about twenty. He kisses me on the neck and moves his hands down my body so softly. He kisses me down to my breasts and parts the chains to get at my nipples.

Sometimes I come at this point while masturbating, but if not, I continue on this line.

I am getting wet, and he pulls away from me and pushes a button on a hand unit, and my legs systematically part. He moves back to me and unhooks the shield on his sexual organ. It is beautiful and not too large. He starts to enter me without removing my pants; then I realize they are crotchless.

I always come by then.

THE MAN is always fantastically built and hung like my lover, who is about seven and a half inches when hard.

Thank you so much, Nancy, for what you are bringing out about our gentler sex. I always thought there was something wrong with me for having these thoughts and masturbating. Love ya and keep up the good work.

Isolde

First off, let me say I have read *My Secret Garden*, and I found it extremely stimulating and full of what the world needs more of—letting men know that we women are really very erotic critters. I've known since I was ten when my fantasy life began—wake up, world!

Before I get into my fantasy life, let me outline my personal reality. I'm twenty-one years old, married, pregnant, a high school graduate, middle class, and, if it's important, white. My husband is twenty-five, one year of college, white, and sexy as hell.

I have been a topless dancer since I was seventeen, and I can't remember a time when I wasn't bisexual—curiously enough, only in reality, never in fantasy. Only sometimes I'll see a sexy girl in *Penthouse* or *Playboy*, and wonder what she'd be like in bed.

I engaged in sexual intercourse for the first time at

thirteen, and have always "played" with myself. I first remember getting caught at five, being told, "Tch, tch, nasty!" I first achieved orgasm at ten. I never came with intercourse until I was fifteen, when a twenty-one-year-old lover taught me the "joy" (God bless him) of oral foreplay.

I have fucked, one way or another, over a hundred men and about thirty women, the first being my cousin, when we were eleven. I guess since I thoroughly enjoy being a topless dancer, you could call me an exhibitionist. And my husband loves to watch me dance. I met him when I was eighteen, and there has never been any hassle about my dancing. He realizes I'm very professional about it, and your typical barroom Joe doesn't turn me on. (We have only been married for eight months.)

My husband has been to bed with over two hundred women, and only one man, a gay mutual friend. Even then, it was at my insistence. Our sexuality, and belief that marriage and personal freedom go hand-in-hand have made us perfect for each other.

When we have intercourse, I always come. If I can't make it during intercourse, which I do ninety percent of the time, we masturbate me after. Sometimes I fuck him in a way he comes quickly, when I know he's horny, and then lay back and enjoy, enjoy!!

Since he's hung pretty heavy, almost nine inches when erect, painful intercourse has always been a problem, and now it's terrible. Being pregnant has made my poor vagina shorter, so careful is the key word. And it's turned me off somewhat.

I have tried to suck him off to make up for my lack of interest. I only succeed in making myself sick. I can't understand it, either, 'cause I love doing it.

There have only been two bad experiences in my sexual life. One was being raped at knife point by a black guy, and being raped anally by a fiancé. I took both in stride, and said fuck it! It doesn't bother me now, except when my husband wants to try anal intercourse. The remembered pain makes me tighten up, and it's impossible.

Our marriage is very open. I have had sexual intercourse, an affair, with one man since becoming pregnant. I guess I was trying to show myself I was still desirable.

We had two threesomes, one where I got all the attention from hubby and hetero friend. In the other, he got the attention from me and a gay friend. I loved it!

I have an active fantasy life. I used to fantasize about raping a guy, sadistically. When we were reading *My Secret Garden,* I asked him about his fantasies. Well, it seems he dug black garter belts and stockings. And being dominated. We went out and bought the necessary articles, and then I dominate him to our hearts' content. I even made him put on the black panties I had on, and then I teased him. I got rough, and made him beg. We loved it! Then I made him eat me, all the time being physically and verbally abusive. The orgasm, when we finally got around to intercourse, was superb.

One of my favorite fantasies is my husband sucking cock. He looked really far out when he had one in his mouth. Sometimes when I masturbate, I picture him making it with a guy, and I come in no time flat!

I also fantasize about being tied spread-eagle on the bed, and my husband playing the domination role to the hilt. I picture him with a huge hard-on, fucking me, and then forcing me to lick him clean of my juices. Then he takes his cock in his hand and slowly starts jacking off, inches from my eyes, telling me what a cunt I am. I try to shut my eyes, but he slaps me and pulls my hair forcing my head back and my mouth open. Suddenly, he stops and tells me he's going to fuck my tits. He pushes my tits together, sucking and biting them. His cock is huge now, and he pushes it up and down, hitting my neck with its head at every thrust. Suddenly, he's sitting with his ass on my tits, and he's jerking his come all over my face, in my eyes, ears, everywhere. I strain to get his cock in my mouth, but he just laughs, keeping it slightly out of reach. (Wow, you don't know what it's doing to me to write this down!)

CHAPTER SEVEN

DURING SEX

☐ Perhaps one sentence I hear more than any other when I am introduced as the author of the book on women's sexual fantasies is, "Oh, I never need fantasies during sex with my husband [lover]. He's all I need. I just think about him, how he feels, etc., etc." I get this response even from women who have read *My Secret Garden* and who must, therefore, know that for every single fantasy sent in by a woman who says she fantasizes during sex, at least two or three were published from women who imagined erotic scenes while walking down the street, masturbating, watching television, and so forth. If I am bored with the stereotyped response that can only see a fantasy taking place during sex, I am nevertheless curious as to why so many women choose to sidestep the question of sexual fantasies by saying their sex is so great they don't "need" them. (Let me hasten to add here that this determination to limit all fantasy as occurring only during sex is very frequent among men too.)

The explanation, I believe, is that none of us want to appear lacking or inadequate in the one area where none of us has absolute, rocklike confidence: our sexuality. We know so little about ourselves that we rush to the defense before anyone has raised a questioning brow. We protest too much; we are afraid to admit we do not have fantasies, because that might be admitting being left out of something. We boast instead that our sex is "great" without it. The entire matter of sexual fantasy is dismissed as being too trivial to discuss. This almost compulsive denial that they "need" fantasy during sex serves two protective functions. First, it denies that you are not woman enough "to do it naturally" (whatever that is). Second, it is a defense against any possible implication that your lover/husband is not enough man.

Most women can only admit to sexual fantasy if it is placed in a lighthearted, nonthreatening context. Show someone an advertisement for a movie with Paul Newman in bed with Ann-Margret. Then suggest to her that a fantasy is merely a little balloon over her head, a little picture of herself taking Ann-Margret's place, if only for an instant. Ah, yes—she will smile—we all get these funny ideas occasionally, don't we?

But ask if she might entertain a fantasy of being in bed with her husband's best friend while he, her husband, is actually fucking her—and all the defenses of heaven and hell break loose. *I am impugning both her and her husband's sexuality!* The thought is so frightening, the consequent angry defense is so overwhelming that how can she admit she has sexual fantasies to me—much less to herself? "When I'm with my husband, we turn each other on so much we don't *need* sexual fantasies, thank you!"

The whole effort is very understandable, and all too human. In the end, I believe the entire confusion grows out of misunderstanding one word: *need.*

What is all this talk of "needing" a fantasy? Do you "need" a martini in those romantic prefucking hours . . . do you "need" that terrific background music . . . do you merely "need" him to put it in and pump away? In all these matters, it's not a question of needing. We try to make an art of lovemaking; a drink, a bit of music are ingredients of the art—*and for many people, so is a sexual fantasy!*

If a sexual fantasy helps turn us on to a higher erotic pitch than we ordinarily reach, it does not mean we are deficient lovers. What it means is that you can't bring up a young woman to say *no, no,* for the first twenty years of her life and then expect her to be able to loosen the grip of habit and repression overnight just because a marriage ceremony has been performed; the sexual brakes are built too deeply into our very nerves, muscles, and blood cells.

In his recent study, *The Female Orgasm,* Dr. Seymour Fisher pinpoints the single greatest reason why so many women are unable to reach orgasm: they are unable "to let go." We have been trained to distrust sexual excitement when we feel it beginning to build up within ourselves; there have been too many warnings about "going too far," and "letting things get out of hand." If something happens, it is the woman's fault—that's the accepted folk wisdom our mothers tried to install in us. We are thus given the responsibility for putting the dampers not only on our own sexuality, but on the man's as well. Is it any surprise that many a woman remains overcontrolled in bed, even when she is there by her own choice, with a man she loves?

Women without number must have discovered on their own, as I did, that sexual fantasies are an almost never-fail method of releasing yourself from a puritanic bondage. You may have intellectually discarded the old sexual rules and inhibitions long ago, but they still grip you emotionally, crippling your sexual response. *This may be true no matter how ardent or skilled your lover may be!* "I have a variety of fantasies which dance through my head on those occasions when I can't seem to get into the sexual act with my lover," writes Lynn. "It has nothing to do with what a great fuck he is, because he is that: fantastic! But sometimes my head just won't turn off everything that's been going on all day. I can't relax, and so I just switch on one of [my fantasies]."

Until the publication of *My Secret Garden,* there had never been any public acknowledgment of the undoubted fact that sexual fantasy was a great aid to female eroticism. It is as if society did not want to grant women so much sexual power, so much erotic self-stimulation. Like so many billions of docile radio or television sets, we were supposed to wait until we had been "turned on" by men.

Unfortunately, women themselves did not help each

other break out of this consipiracy of silence; it left us passive victims of the male mystique of what sex was. We did not feel free enough to discuss our sexual fantasies and ideas even with our best friends (until only the most recent years).

Thus, each woman was left feeling isolated, guilty, and alone with her sexual fantasies . . . convinced she was some kind of freak or pervert if she entertained or enjoyed these ideas. Her husband or lover had never mentioned having any sexual fantasies himself; nor in his idle talk about the women he knew before her (to which she listened more carefully than he knew) did she ever pick up the slightest clue that other women had sexual fantasies like hers. ". . . I am writing this almost stealthily," says Jan, after an unflinching catalog of some of the most erotic fantasies in this book, "as I would be embarrassed at being discovered. . . . I was never able to be very open about sex, because my husband . . . is the romantic sort, and believes very much in the sanctity of marriage." While she feels stimulated by X-rated films, she can't go to them, because her husband doesn't approve. "Some of my fantasies are very similar to those of the other women that you published," she finishes her letter. "I guess we are not alone no matter how bizarre we think our own are."

"Your book was excellent," writes Kate. "I thought my fantasies were abnormal, and I felt very guilty about them. Now I realize almost everyone has them."

It is time for this kind of unnecessary guilt to stop, for women to realize that no matter how extraordinary the sexual events they like to imagine that increase their passion while in bed with their lovers, they are not alone. □

Lynn

I have a variety of fantasies which dance through my head on those occasions when I can't seem to get into the sexual act with my lover. It has nothing to do with what a great fuck he is, because he is that: fantastic! But sometimes my head just won't turn off everything that's been going on all day, I can't relax, and so I just switch on one of the following:

Fantasy 1: I am having sex with two guys, neither of whom is my lover. They are both going down on me simultaneously. This may sound impossible, but the one kind of acts like relief man for the other, so that the rhythm never stops, and they are both insatiable. I should add that I take a long time to come, so having two men relieves me of worrying about one of them getting tired.

Fantasy 2: Sometimes when my lover is in the mood and I'm kind of distracted, we leave the television on with the sound turned off. I make sure there's a channel turned on with at least one terrific-looking man, and then while we're making love, I like to think that he and everyone else on the show are watching *our* act and loving it.

Fantasy 3: I will close my eyes and imagine a crowd, maybe on the street, in a store, even a crowd at a party. The whole group is fascinated watching me masturbate, watching the beautiful expressions on my face. Eventually, they all begin to masturbate too.

Fantasy 4: I often fantasize this on my way to work as well as during sex: that I am on a crowded bus, and, without anyone minding or exclaiming, I just reach down inside this good-looking guy's trousers and masturbate him. All the while, he's standing there, holding on to the strap and going weak in the knees as I bring him closer and closer to climax. He never looks at me, but I know he is just praying I won't stop. If I am sitting in front of him in my fantasy, I will often lean forward and put his prick in my mouth just before he comes.

Fantasy 5: Very often the men in my fantasies are strangers. More often than not. I find it terribly exciting if, while they are fucking me, they also use the most profane language imaginable. I don't really like men to whisper words in my ear while we're really fucking; somehow it seems so fake. But the strangers in my fantasies know just how to use these words, and not only is there no embarrassment, but it is madly exciting. For instance, they say things like. "My cock is in your cunt, and it's on fire. . . ." "I want to come all over you, in your ears, in your ass, etc."

I don't always use these fantasies, but they sure help me forget about the problems of the day when I want to pay all my attention to sex and just relax and get into it.

Good luck and please understand that I really do love my man. . . . It's just that the fantasies help me love him more.

Jan

Happily married for many years to a lusty man, and having borne several children, nevertheless, I had not experimented with any kinky sex, mainly because of my husband's innocence of such things. An early fantasy I would employ during sex to further stimulate myself would be that I was an innocent young girl propositioned by a sensuous older man. I would be kept by him in great luxury (this was during a time in real life when we were quite desperately poor) in return for a surrender of my virginity and the willingness to submit to his every whim. I agree, and he deflowers me on an obstetrical table, with my feet in stirrups.

After the initial loss of my cherry, he proceeds to teach me exactly what to do, and arouses me with aphrodisiacs, so that I am dripping and begging for him to fuck me. He has me walk on all fours and beg like a dog for it. He sadistically makes me wait and suffer mightily until he satisfies my lust.

After several months, he is satisfied that I am properly trained, and he take me to a secret place—a huge manor house somewhere (afterward, when I read the *Story of O* . . . it sounded so similar) when I am told that I will be on exhibition for members of his club, a club devoted to eroticism and sensuality.

251

Other girls and I are kept naked and chained in cages part of the day, while the club members examine us like animals in a zoo. At mealtime, we are the waitresses, and submit to being fondled and roughly inspected internally as well as externally. We are told to bend over to pick up a purposely dropped spoon, and fingers are then inserted into our cunts.

Breasts are weighed and measured, rulers inserted into cunts, and sizes recorded. We find out why that evening.

There is a special show, an exhibition of the specialties of the various girls and their "benefactors." The men sit in a circle around a stage, and the show begins. A tiny girl no bigger than a child is led in, followed by a huge black man. His penis is enormous. It turns out that she has systematically been enlarged by the insertion of bigger and bigger dildos, and now they are putting her to the test. But no, it is still too big, and she writhes in pain. Finally, he succeeds, and with her legs around his waist, he manipulates her against him.

The next act is a huge cow of a woman, with udderlike breasts and a huge bouncy ass. She does a dance for her audience, and everything shakes like jelly. Her cunt is enormous, and, therefore, two little men, dwarfs almost, come in and both penetrate her at the same time. Every expression on her face is mirrored in the eyes of the watching men. When she comes, she bellows like a cow.

By this time, having fantasized all this, I am usually really aroused, and often didn't finish the fantasy. I never get the chance to perform with my specialty.

Now, years later, having started to educate myself with the *Sensuous Woman,* followed by some of the more readily available erotic classics, my fantasies have changed somewhat. Now I employ group scenes, myself and another woman, and other kinky combinations. Recently, we (my husband and I) went to see the *Devil and Miss Jones,* and I was partially repelled by seeing everything I'd read about in privacy in giant living color, but at the same time, I was fascinated, and the impressions stayed with me for weeks afterward.

Actually, I am writing this almost stealthily, as I would be embarrassed at being discovered, therefore, all the typing errors.

I was never able to be very open about sex, because my husband, although having a large carnal appetite, is the romantic sort and believes very much in the sanctity of marriage, and doesn't care for the X-rated films. He says he won't go again. It did stimulate me very much, and I would love to go again, provided it was a well-made film.

One of my present fantasies is ticked off when I see a local girl at the supermarket. She isn't beautiful, but somehow I am aroused by her. I imagine her naked, and I am caressing her. (I do this while caressing myself.) She never wears a bra, and I always notice dark nipples under her clothing. This titillates me. Her breasts are large, and I love to play with them in my fantasy. I don't like to go down on her, but I do finger her cunt and fuck her with a large dildo. I sometimes drive her wild with a vibrator. I get a double dildo and slide it into both openings. She moans with delight and throws her body around and trembles uncontrollably. At this point in my imaginings, I come.

A fantasy I employ when my husband and I are making it is that we are the center of attention at a large orgy in a sultan's opulent palace. The sultan is watching to make sure that his women are working properly. I must lift my ass high off the bed, or I will be punished. The punishment is being fucked in the ass by a large dog. At this point, I usually come.

Some of my fantasies are very similar to those of the other women that you published. I guess we are not alone no matter how bizarre we think our own are. Thank you for a needed research. I hope that I may have been of some help.

Isabel

I purchased *My Secret Garden* yesterday, and have completed reading it already. Needless to say, I found it fascinating and very enlightening.

I'm a twenty-four-year-old married woman. My husband is also twenty-four, and we have no children. We have a fairly good sex life. (We have been married three years.) I'm not what you'd call pretty. I'm average-looking and slightly overweight (fifteen pounds). My husband is fairly good-looking and about ten pounds overweight.

Last year, during our lovemaking, I just stopped reaching climax, although I'd had no trouble before then. My doctor can find no physical reason for this. Now, the only way I can achieve orgasm is to fantasize during our lovemaking.

I know my husband sometimes fantasizes about other women, because he's told me he has. Part of the problem may be because he is fairly quiet during lovemaking, while I'm pretty noisy—moans, etc. I perform fellatio on him, and sometimes he performs oral sex on me, but not as often or as long as I'd like him to. I've told him this, but he ignores it. I really enjoy doing oral sex on him.

Well, this fantasy I have is about ice hockey players. We live in a city with a professional team, and I've always liked the sport since I was a teenager. My husband doesn't care for any other sport except hockey. I've talked to some of the players. What I fantasize about during our lovemaking is about these players, and the uglier-looking they are, the better I like them.

My fantasy begins with me in the locker room. Of course, I'm all dressed up in an attractive pant-suit, makeup, and my hair has just been done. There's a table there, sort of like the kind doctors use to examine people. Maybe it's the one players use when they get a rub-down. The players come in and ask me what I'm doing there. I make up a story, saying I'm writing a story on them for the newspaper.

They start taking off their equipment and skates, acting like I'm just another one of the guys. Then my very favorite player, still in his uniform, comes over to me and gives me the "once over" look. He asks me to go out with him after his shower and change. I confess to him that I've always wanted to have sex with him. He seems pleased, since he's a single, swinging-type. He walks me over to the table and says, "How about now?" I protest because there are the other players around. In fact, they are watching and listening while pretending not to, and now my favorite player tells them what I just said. They laugh and make comments, but really, I know they envy him.

As long as I've gone this far, I go ahead and tell them that some of them are men I would like to have sex with too. Not all of them, but only certain ones and in a certain order. My favorite is the biggest man on the team, very masculine and ugly, with hockey scars on his cheek. I place the others in a descending order of size and this certain kind of mean look. Some of the players on my list are married, but they are very hot for me and never dream of saying no to being on my list. (Naturally, in a fantasy, no one can refuse me.)

The rest of the players go ahead with whatever they were doing. The ones I chose stand by the table, waiting their turn, and telling each other how lucky they are to have sex with a beautiful woman like me. Sometimes they say that my few extra pounds are exactly what they like, that it makes me more of a woman. Other times, I imagine myself to be more slender than I really am, with a body that drives these men wild.

My favorite, first choice then approaches me, and slowly strips me under the overhead light that hangs over the rubbing-down table. He's kissing me all over and telling me how much he likes my large breasts. (My husband is a breast freak—the larger the better.) By this time, I'm feeling all those hungry eyes that I did not choose watching me enviously from the darkness as they slowly go on changing their clothes, but I'm also getting turned on by the feel of my favorite, who has been slowly taking off his uniform all the while. He is on top of me, caressing and kissing me all over, especially my breasts —which turns me on in reality just as it does in fantasy. Then, while the waiting players are all watching, and I can see them growing erect themselves as they wait their turn, my favorite slowly goes down on me, eating me until I'm writhing with pleasure. The next man in line can't wait, and while the first player has his face buried between my legs, the second man is licking my nipples. The two feelings at once, a tongue between my legs and another licking and sucking my nipples has me in such a frenzy that I come—without knowing which man has made it happen. But I can't even think about that because almost with a shock of happy surprise, before I am even out of orgasm, I realize that the first man has moved his body up higher, and he is fucking me. I feel his hard-on pumping up inside me like some kind of great, powerful machine, his balls banging up against the backs of my thighs and asshole as he lunges deeper and deeper into me. I tell him how big he is and how good all that bigness feels inside me and for him not to stop. I like the way he laughs a little right here in my fantasy and says for me not to worry, he won't stop until he's done—which takes a long time.

(My husband doesn't take a very long time to reach orgasm, which often leaves me feeling unsatisfied.)

The player then tells me how much he enjoyed eating me and how much it turned him on. Now it is the turn of the other players, starting with the man who was licking my nipples. He has an erection that is so big and painful, he has to hold it in his hands, rubbing it to soothe the ache. When I open my legs for him, he rams it in so fast and hard he almost pushes me off the table. Starting with him, each man doesn't take very long to come. They are barely inside me when with a wriggle of my hips, and a squeeze of my inside muscles, I milk them, and they come in a big explosion. I don't care because I want them to come quickly, I want to feel how fast

I can make a man come and besides, as soon as one man is finished, there is another one on line to step forward and begin to fuck me as if the last man had not yet stopped.

I tell them all how good each one is, and they tell me how good I am. Also, while they fuck me, they're noisy about it. I love to hear their groans, shouts of impatience, and, above all, their obscenities like, "I'm gonna fuck the hell out of you," etc.

Of course, I have to really imagine each one nude and what they'd look like, but I have practice in this, because I like to imagine them naked while they are skating and playing their hockey game, so by the time they enter into this fantasy, I have already thought up how they look, and I am almost "at home" with their nakedness.

After they have all had a turn—they have only fucked me, only the first player, my favorite, went down on me—I turn back to him, my first choice. I tell him he's so good that I am dying for another fuck. He's very pleased because he's so good at it. He moves me forward to the edge of the table, so that my hips are almost off the edge. In this way, he can fuck me standing up. I wrap my legs around his hips to hold him close to me, and he slowly puts his arms up over his head, like a prizefighter who has just won the fight—all the while continuing to pump away inside me. "Go to it!" "That's it—fuck her good!" all the other players are cheering him on, but he and I know without saying it that he wouldn't be this good—certainly not this second time in such a short space of time—with any other woman but me. This time, he comes while I watch him. He just groans as if his last breath is escaping him, and he slumps down and falls across my stomach. He's out, and all the players are crowding around me, kissing me, telling me how great I am, what a woman I am, etc.

I also use this fantasy when I masturbate, since I can change the players and make them do anything to me I want. (Except I don't fantasize anal penetration, because I don't think I'd care for it.) I really get turned on thinking about having sex with these guys who are so big. The only time I masturbate is after I'm left frustrated when my husband doesn't give me an orgasm. I've got pictures of some of the players, including my favorite, and I look at them and close my eyes while I masturbate with the smooth, rounded handle of a hairbrush. I can *always* give myself an orgasm.

My husband doesn't know I masturbate, but I think maybe he might get turned on if he ever did watch me. Once, he made me rub my own breasts while he watched and got turned on. He was fingering me at the time. I didn't like doing it myself. I'd rather have him rub me.

That's my fantasy. I can't help but have it flash through my mind at least briefly whenever we go to a hockey game. My husband knows I like some of the players, and he sort of goes along with it sometimes. Like a couple of times, when we were making love, he'd say, "I'm—(player's name), and I want to fuck you, baby." He does this becuase part of him knows this turns me on, and he enjoys my excitement, but part of him doesn't really like it, that it is the idea of the other man that is getting me so excited—even though my husband himself is the one who brings the other man to my mind.

Thank you for reading this letter. I hope it didn't sound too weird! It's similar to some of the ones I read in your book, except my fantasy *isn't* a gang-rape fantasy. It's one guy at a time, and they aren't forcing me to do anything. In fact, I have chosen them and make each one wait his turn till I'm ready for him.

Maybe if you write another book, you could use this fantasy. I'd be thrilled to see it in print, being read by millions (maybe) of people, who wouldn't know it was me. (Please *don't* use my real name.)

P.S. If my fantasy ever does happen in reality, It'd be interesting to see a player going down on me since all my favorite players have rather large noses.

Kate

Your book was excellent. I thought my fantasies were abnormal, and I felt very guilty about them. Now I realize almost everyone has them.

I am twenty, well educated, and well traveled. I have been married less than two months. My husband and I both used to use drugs heavily, but now we only smoke pot once in a while. I tell you this because I think that drugs and smoking help a great deal to heighten awareness of your fantasies.

One night recently, I seemed to be taking too long to come, so I started fantasizing. (This is the first time I remember doing it during sex.) It had a remarkable effect on arousing me. I fantasized that I was a prostitute—well, not exactly a prostitute, but a woman with nothing to lose by fucking every man she wanted —and I was out to fuck every man in town. As I fantasized, my whole body began to feel like it was being fucked by every man imaginable; there wasn't a shred of me that wasn't being aroused by some man. I got off better than I ever had before with my husband or the five other lovers I have had.

Another fantasy I have is that my ex-lovers are all doing me at once, each doing the thing he did best. However, my favorite fantasy, the one I use mostly now (and find the most erotic), is that I am tied up, and a gang of rapists are making me fuck a dog. They are all watching me and all getting hard-ons and waiting to fuck me themselves once I come with the dog. The dog is licking my clitoris, and I am made to perform fellatio on the dog. Soon the dog and I are both getting out of control as we both want more and more. We both come at the same time. Then the dog fucks me. All of my moaning has made the men even more aroused. Then they each take turns, doing what the dog did. Each one is hornier than the next, and each one is a better fuck. I come with all of them. I think that seeing me fuck that dog aroused those men more than any sight imaginable.

I should mention that I was once raped. So that the idea of this last fantasy really happening disgusts me. Actually, after I was raped, I was violently ill; it happened in an alley, and I remember vomiting after they left me. I never hitchhike anymore or even walk at night without my husband, unless it's down a well-lit street. My favorite pastimes used to be walking in the country, the mountains, or the woods, just getting off by myself, but now I wouldn't dare. If I must walk alone, I carry something that could be used as a weapon. I always thought I'd never be able to kill a person, but if an attacker should ever approach me again, I wouldn't hesitate to maim or kill him. When you are 4′ 11″ and 86 pounds you need protection.

I suppose you wonder how I could be so aroused by this last fantasy, given what has happened to me. It makes me wonder too. The best idea I can come up with is that the dog is the best fucker in the group . . . no man can top him. I'm not *really* angry at men, certainly not my husband, but I guess there's some anger left over somewhere. Anyway, the fantasy does the trick for me, and that's all that matters.

☐ In Kate's fantasy, which appears immediately above, I am very impressed by the self-analysis that she gives us at the end of her note. As we have seen in many other women's letters, the seeds of the fantasy that she seems to tell with the most relish and erotic excitement were sown in an actual, horrible event. She was raped. "I always thought I'd never be able to kill a person," she writes, "but if an attacker should ever approach me again, I wouldn't hesitate to maim or kill him." Her murderous feelings are still unappeased in real life, but by an imaginative use of fantasy, she has found some place to put this anger so that it does not come between her and her husband. Her fantasy turns the tables on the men who raped and humiliated her, and expresses a kind of exquisite sexual revenge: she would rather fuck a dog than any of them. "I'm not *really* angry at men," she writes, "certainly not my husband, but I guess [the rape left] some anger left over somewhere." This anger is expressed and used up in fantasy, even while having sex with her husband. Whether he knows or not, he is as much the gainer as she is. "The fantasy does the trick for me," she happily concludes, "and that's all that matters."

Neither Helen nor Riva have to keep their sexual fantasies hidden from their husbands. Helen's fantasy, in fact, was originally invented by her husband for the two of them to share. While it is all about him assisting while she is fucked by another man, Helen credits the excitement this idea brings to their bedroom as one of the prime ingredients of a "wonderfully happy and successful marriage" of many years. Her husband, Helen says, "is the most wonderful, kind, thoughtful, considerate and lusty man any woman could ever hope to have for her own."

Riva also finds that talking about her fantasies during sex adds to the spice and erotic satisfactions of her eight-year-old marriage. But while Helen and her husband say they would now like to find a man to act out their fantasy with them, Riva has no such idea. "I have never done any of these things," she writes, "and have really no desire to even see them happen in real life . . . too scared, I guess . . . but they make great conversation in bed and make me wild with my husband, usually bringing him to come at the climax of the fantasy."

How wise both husbands sound to me. They do not see the imaginary lovers who heat their wives' sexual imagination as impossible rivals, but as sexual assistants instead, who help each man bring his wife to the kind of excitement that makes marriage alive and tingling.

While Beth too shares her fantasies aloud with her husband, there is a variation. The fantasy he likes to hear most is about his wife making love to another woman.

"Paul likes me to talk about this during sex," Beth writes, "but not any other time." But since Beth writes that she is the mother of two children, "married and very happy and contented," isn't that their business? Fantasies work for some people in one way; they work for others in a different one. If yours works for you, isn't that all that really matters? □

Helen

My husband and I have just finished reading *My Secret Garden,* and we both enjoyed it so much that I feel it is only fair that I write to tell you about our favorite fantasy.

I say "our" because this was originally my husband's fantasy. But he has told it to me so many times, and he is so excited by the idea (and has made me so excited by it), that it has become my favorite fantasy as well.

If you are interested in background; my husband is a virile, horny fifty-six years of age. He is a college graduate with a post-graduate degree in business administration. I am an eager and receptive forty-eight, and a graduate of commercial college. We have had a wonderfully happy and successful marriage for twenty-five years. We have two fine sons, one of whom is in his first year of post-graduate work, and the other in his third year of undergraduate study. My husband has said many times that I am as close as God ever came to making a perfect woman, and as gorgeous a piece of ass as he's ever seen. And I think he is the most wonderful, kind, thoughtful, considerate, and lusty man any woman could ever hope to have for her own. We both agree that our delightfully happy sex life is a prime ingredient of our wonderfully successful marriage.

My husband's (and mine) most exciting fantasy is to have another man join us in our sexual recreation. Every time we see an attractive, virile-looking man, we speculate as to whether he might be the one we are searching for.

In our fantasy, my imaginary lover lies on his back (we are all three naked, of course) while I kneel astride his head so he can eat my pussy to get it ready for his cock. Meanwhile, my husband lies between my lover's legs and sucks his cock to get it ready for my pussy.

When I am warm and wet and my lover is hot and hard, I move down and kneel astride his hips. With one hand, my husband opens my pussy lips and with the other, he guides my lover's cock into me. Then he lays between my lover's legs and watches as I slide my streaming pussy up and down the full length of that hard throbbing shaft.

Slowly and teasingly, I raise up until my husband can see my lover's strained, purplish cockhead nestled between the soft, wet lips of my pussy. Then I slowly sink down and take the full length of that hard, hot shaft into me right up to the balls.

After every ten or twelve strokes, I lift completely off my lover's prick so my husband can take it in his mouth. He says the idea of tasting my pussy juice on another man's cock just drives him wild.

We keep up this slow, teasing stroking of his straining shaft by my pussy, alternating with sucking by my husband, until my poor imaginary lover can stand it no longer. Lying between his legs, my husband holds my lover's balls while he explodes and his bursting cock squirts a torrent of thick, rich, hot cream into the depths of my hungry cunt. I continue to stroke his cock with my pussy until I have sucked him dry of the last drops of his cream, and his cock shrivels and drops out of me. Immediately, I roll over on my back beside him and spread my legs wide to receive my ravenous husband. In one bound, he is between my eager thighs, and one thrust buries his lovely, hard cock in me right up to the balls.

He is excited beyond description to feel how slick and slippery I am from the tremendous load of sperm that another man's cock has just pumped into my cunt. He says nothing is as exciting as to be able to feel another man's cream in my cunt while he fucks me.

He is too excited to last very long while we act out this fantasy, and it is never more than a minute or two before I feel his beloved cock jumping and jerking in my cunt as his hot sperm gushes into my belly in a flood of molten fire. In my own fantasy, I feel my husband's sperm mixing inside me with my lover's sperm until my cunt overflows, and I feel their mingled cream running down the crack of my ass to puddle warmly and soothingly beneath me. At that point, I join my husband in a gut-twisting orgasm that leaves us both too exhausted to move. Until ten or fifteen minutes, that is. Then we're ready for No. 2.

Someday we hope to find a real life lover who will be interested in joining us, so that we can act out in actuality our favorite fantasy of having another man put his cock in me and cream my cunt before my husband fucks me.

P.S. I knew my husband would enjoy reading this (I had told him I intended to write you), so after I had finished typing it, I went up to the bedroom, took off my bra and panties, and came down to the living room dressed in just a skirt and blouse.

As he read, I saw that delightful bulge beginning to rise in his pants. I hurried to kneel between his legs, pulled down his zipper, took out his beautiful cock, and lovingly sucked it up to its full, seven-and-one-half-inch towering height of stiff male meat. I was careful not to bring him off in my mouth, because I wanted to share with him the delight of once again acting out our favorite fantasy.

When he had finished reading my letter, I looked up at him and asked in my most pleading, little-girl voice, "Can we pretend my fantasy lover has just skewered me on his prick and emptied his balls into my belly, and my cunt is dripping wet with his hot, slippery sperm? I want to get fucked."

And I did, most satisfactorily. With his hands trembling in his excitement and eagerness, my husband stripped off my blouse and skirt, laid me down on the floor, dropped his pants, and fell to his knees between my wide spread thighs. I took his magnificent stiff, throbbing cock in my hand, guided it lovingly into my ravennous cunt, and moaned in ecstasy as he buried it in me up to the balls, and frantically fucked me into a glorious orgasm. Right in the middle of the living-room floor.

If every married couple found in their sexual relations the joy and delight that my husband and I have shared for twenty-five years, divorce would be as dead as the dinosaurs. In opening the door to a frank discussion of the subject of sexual fantasies, which add so much spice to the sexual act itself, you have contributed immeasurably toward that end, and we think you have richly earned the appreciation and congratulations of everybody who has the intelligence to read your book and the courage to act out and enjoy her own fantasies.

Riva

Just finished reading *My Secret Garden* . . . fascinating! Of course, when I saw your address, I just couldn't resist writing. I am twenty-six and have been married for eight years. My husband is from India. I first started fantasizing at his request, after we were married about five years. It really livened things up. He enjoys it a great deal when I swear during the sex act—I don't normally at other times. Using very filthy language, I describe various situations he would probably enjoy seeing me in.

One is that I am a prostitute, and I am working for him. He is able to see all my actions from behind a two-way mirror. I proceed to suck a customer and kiss his balls, and it all really drives him crazy. Then he fucks me, or if I am sucking him, he squirts his semen all over my face.

Another is that I am being fucked by two guys while my husband is watching. One is shoving his cock down my throat, and the other is sucking my cunt. My breasts are also being massaged. I can't move because of the size of the cock going down my throat. The two guys agree to come at the same time, so simultaneously, one goes off in my cunt, and the other in my mouth, which I proceed to suck and swallow in great gulps.

Another fantasy is that of being gang raped by a motorcycle gang or of being *initiated* into the gang. When I am initiated, one guy must screw me, and I must go down on each one of them. Also the girls must go down on me until I come with each one. In the rape scene, I am tied down to the bed and cannot move. One guy forces his cock in my mouth, another one performs cunnilingus on me, and he sucks my tits. At the same time, another bastard sticks a dildo or vibrator up my asshole. Again I cannot scream or fight. Gradually, I become ecstatic, and the guy doing the lick job puts his cock in me and blows off. This is repeated with members of the gang, and of course, I am so hot I am going crazy.

Another fantasy is one of fucking with a friend or a guy at work. My husband wants to hear all the details of every situation. Another is one of me and another girl pleasing my husband, and also him pleasing me. I think of him licking me out while he fucks her and vice versa.

I could go on and on, as I am always making up new and varied situations (especially after getting new ideas from your book). I have never done any of these things and have really no desire to even see them happen in real life . . . too scared, I guess . . . but they make great conversation in bed and make me wild with my husband, usually bringing him to come at the climax of the fantasy.

Beth

I have just this minute finished reading *My Secret Garden*, and am I glad I read it! Now I know that I'm not the only one who makes up stories. I'm writing this to tell you some of my own fantasies.

I'm nineteen, with two children, married, and very happy and contented. My husband is twenty-four, and we are middle- to upper-middle-class whites. My oldest child is a boy, the other a girl.

One fantasy I've just recently realized is about my husband's car. I knew there had to be a reason why I liked to drive it so much. It's a '67 Camaro, very fast, and sexy. It's a manual transmission, which is the object of my fantasy. The gearshift is between the bucket seats on the console and has a big smooth knob which I love to caress as I'm driving. The motions necessary to shift gears plus the speed is fantastic. I'm ready for sex in no time.

Another one is from an actual incident. My husband took me to a party at a friend's mobile home. This was a year before we married and a month after we met. Besides him, I only knew Dave, his best friend, and Celeste, his sister. Dave and Celeste have slept together on occasion. My husband got involved in a game of Euchre and the three of us were left to talk. I drank quite a bit of beer, and after a while, Dave took us in the bedroom, where the coats were, to show us a chain he had made from beer pop-top rings. I noticed some paperbacks (pornography) on the dresser and opened one at random and began to read aloud. We sat on the bed, and when I came to a part that said, "and she kissed his ear following with her tongue and warm, moist breath," I leaned over to Dave and did what I just read. So did Celeste on his other ear. He alternated kissing us both, and that is where it ended, as we were interrupted with some fat jerk yelling, "Hey, they're having an orgy in here!" I like to fantasize what might have happened if we hadn't been interrupted . . . Dave making slow, exciting love to both of us. Me and Celeste getting it on. We both are large busted and have long dark hair and wear glasses with similar shaped frames. Practically twins . . .

One fantasy I have quite often is about myself, my husband, and another girl. He would bring her home one night, and I'd be there in a flowing gown. I'd kiss and embrace them both, and we'd head right for the bedroom. After much kissing, exploring, and foreplay, Paul would make love to her, after which I'd go down on her to lick up both of their juices and make her come a second time. Paul would be kissing and fondling both of our breasts. Then he would make love to me, after which she'd go down on me, and we would just make love until dawn, take a shower together and sleep all day exhausted. I usually come during the part where I go down on her.

I feel I should tell you that my only experiences have been with men. I never thought of another girl until my husband brought it up during sex one time after we were married. Now I realize that girls do turn me on, and I'd like to be able to have the last fantasy acted out. I guess I'm what they call a bisexual. Paul likes me to talk about this during sex, but not any other time. I also love to have these fantasies during sex. However, he gives me strange looks when I comment on a girl's body and then start giving out horny signals when we're out somewhere. Oh, well, he'll get used to it. Girl's bodies turn him on, too.

Well, thanks so much for doing this. I can't tell anyone else, not even Paul, except the last one. But only during sex.

"Shoulders"

I guess when you say "anonymity guaranteed," you anticipate your letters will come with names on them, but I honestly would not be able to write you if I had to sign this. I hope that doesn't make my "material" less useful.

I have had other, rather mundane fantasies, but through the years (I am twenty-three), they have fallen by the wayside because of the dominance of the one I will describe in this letter. One of the odd things (or is it?) about my fantasy is that it is interchangeable among males, that is the identity of the particular man who plays the leading role in it at any given time is not important. (I am sure you know what "important" means in a fantasy!) Of course, I vary the men to avoid monotony.

The key to the beginning of the fantasy is when the man (or boy!) put his hands on my shoulders. There is usually a build-up to this situation of varying length, but the point when the fantasy takes on seductive and exciting overtones is when I feel his hands on my shoulders. All that really happens is that he forces me to kneel by putting pressure on my shoulders, and then I kiss and suck him down there. He doesn't have to tell me what to do, or even push my head; all communication of what he wants is through that pressure on my shoulders. At the moment of climax for me, the pressure becomes very intense and objectively painful, although not discomforting. I guess since I control my fantasy, I increase the pressure, keeping it in synchronization with my body's excitement. In reality, I have even taken to sort of hunching my shoulders at climax. Luckily, this doesn't seem to bother my partner during intercourse.

I don't know what you can make of this, but I do hope it is useful to you.

☐ Many of the women in this book have talked about fantasy during oral sex. Monica writes that she and her fiancé have sex "quite often seven or eight times a night." But while she describes him as sexually large and powerful, the way he "always brings me to a glorious climax," she writes, is "usually through cunnilingus."

I think this is one of the more obvious times for fantasy

to fill the minds of women like Monica, because in a sense you are passive, the recipient, being done to. Your body is not being covered by and entwined with another body . . . your eyes are not looking into a beloved face but into space. For many women, fantasy fills in what might otherwise be a kind of loneliness during oral sex.

This kind of lovemaking often comes as a later, liberated step for many women. They have resisted oral sex earlier in their sexual lives, before they grew confident enough to become experimental. Perhaps they felt that it was "wrong," or that there is something malodorous or unattractive about themselves "down there." What a sexual fantasy can do for women with these negative ideas is *drive them out*, replacing them with erotic emotions that enable women to enjoy themselves to the full.

Other women have come to oral sex from the opposite extreme—they enjoy it so much that they never want it to end, and through certain sexual fantasies, they have found they can prolong their period of foreplay excitement before reaching climax. This *enhancement* role of fantasy, either during oral sex or intercourse itself, is a valuable idea for those women who experience no trouble in reaching or enjoying their orgasm; knowing they will arrive in due time, they like to imagine a mental scenario that helps them enjoy the trip even more. They pace their excitement in their minds, letting their motor slowly build up speed until it gloriously runs away with them toward an ever more heightened orgasm. Needless to say, these are the women who have long got past the idea that thinking of a man different from the one in their arms smacks of mental adultery or betrayal; they have recognized that their own excitement, no matter how it is achieved, is one of the greatest sexual gifts they can bring a man.

I have always maintained that women are experts at fantasy. It is a natural gift that most of us have denied ourselves simply because, in a man's world, it was "known" that men . . . and therefore *everybody* . . . did not fantasize during sex. Today, we hear more and more reports of the growing rate of impotency among men. If women can in time learn to accept their gift for fantasy, can we not also teach this form of erotic excitement to our men—probably now at the very time when they need it most? If it works for us, why shouldn't it work for them?

Sexual fantasy during sex is not merely a matter of need. It is a matter of more complete sex. Would you consider a part of your body untouchable during sex? Why then rule out your mind—which is what got you into bed with that specific other person in the first place? A man will not propose sex to a woman unless he is already aroused; it is his fantasy of being in bed with her that has brought him to the point of beginning the seduction. Having been brought to sex by his fantasy, why leave out your own? □

Monica

I've just finished *My Secret Garden,* and all I can say is "what a trip." I just couldn't put it down; it had me creaming from cover to cover.

I don't think I ever realized just how big a part of my sex life fantasy actually was. I have had a fairly active sex life since the time I was sixteen. I am twenty now and about to be married. My first sexual experience was with my furture husband in the back seat of a '62 Chevy. Needless to say, it wasn't the fireworks I expected. But it has been getting better all the time.

My fiancé is hung quite well, as his full erection measures a good—and I mean good—eight inches. We have sex quite often when we are together—very often seven or eight times a night. His imagination is limitless, and he always brings me to a glorious climax, usually through cunnilingus. Although I have been dating him for five years, my sex life has been punctuated with a few, very interesting affairs. It is these affairs that I find myself fantasizing about most—and always during intercourse with my fiancé.

The most remarkable lover in my life came along when I was seventeen years old. He was a phys. ed. teacher, and we worked together during the summer. I just came everytime I thought of his godlike black body. Just looking at him made me wet and achy for his cock. I had never experienced such a feeling before, and I was completely overwhelmed. When the occasion finally came when we could be alone, I was so shaky my knees gave out. He was so gentle and satisfying with his foreplay, I reached several climaxes while he manipulated my clitoris. And when he entered me from the rear—I just saw stars. He filled me up so much I thought I would burst from sheer ecstasy. As we weren't using any birth control, he withdrew, and I sucked him off. When we reached our final climax, he came with such a groan, it heightened my pleasure immensely. I got such a mouthful of his wonderful come that I felt it was Christmas. This was the only time we ever fucked, and I feel it's better that way.

I think of this glorious black man often when I am going down on my fiancé's beautiful rod, as it heightens the pleasure I am able to give him. I merely think of that black cock filling my mouth, and we come off in great fervor.

Please excuse the sloppiness of this letter, as I am masturbating and cannot take the time to recopy it as I fear exposure.

Thanks for the wonderful book.

Delia

I would like to compliment you on your book entitled *My Secret Garden*. It is about time that men are no longer protected! Women think about sex also!

I was pleased to realize that women had fantasies such as mine. I never thought myself to be strange, but I wondered what other women thought about. I found it very interesting and sometimes exciting. I have two fantasies that I would like to share with you. I hope that after reading them you will enjoy them as much as I do.

I imagine that I am in jail, and I am put in a cell of lesbians. The "queen" lesbian decides I need training in female love, so she takes me on as her private student. This all takes place in her cell, with the other women watching. She tells me to undress, and she admires my body. She tells me how beautiful it is, and what she is going to do to me. She then undresses herself and tells me to suck her tits. I am apprehensive at first, but I catch on quickly. After I suck her tits, I work my way down to her cunt. The fantasy is so strong, that I can even smell her odor. I suck her clit and finger her ass, and she explodes in my mouth. Then it is my turn. She works on my clit, and as I am about to come, I beg to get fucked. At the right moment, she shoves this dildo in my cunt, at which point I actually do come. I change the fantasy around, but this is the basic plot.

I have had quite a few lovers in my life, but two stand out. Robert and Henry. They were built like brick shit houses, and they play a large part in my fantasies. My current lover is a novice, so he has a long way to come. (No pun intended.) I can't wait for the day when I tell him about my fantasies. I'm dying to tell him now, but he couldn't accept it. While I am making love to him, if I am on top, I have the following fantasy.

I imagine that I am impaled on Henry's cock, and Robert is easing his cock in my asshole. When I am completely filled in and starting to move, a faceless woman walks in. She fondles my tits and rubs my clitty. At this point, I am jumping around, almost going out of my head. I just concentrate on what they are doing to me, and I have one of my strongest orgasms. Then, of course, I come back into reality, and it's funny. My real lover thinks that he sent me into outer space, while I know for fact, it was my imaginary three. Oh, well.

Thank you for letting me express myself.

Daisy

I'm sending you two of my many sexual fantasies. I am twenty-one and am black. I went to various religious schools and am a college graduate. I moved to California in 1972, and now live there with my fiancé, a gorgeous blond with green eyes and a fantastic body. I was prompted to send you my fantasies after reading your book. Here goes.

Fantasy 1: I fantasize that this really great-looking guy (he's white) kidnaps two high school girls. One is black, and one is white. The black girl is very pretty. She has small breasts and a neat slim figure. She's rather innocent and a virgin. The white girl is a pretty blonde with big breasts and an overall voluptuous figure. The man tells them that he wants to make love to the pretty black girl and that if she doesn't consent he'll have her friend subjected to a very brutal sexual routine. The girl refuses. He calls in five men and have them strip the white girl. He turns to the black girl and tells her that he's going to let the men have her to do with as they please if she doesn't consent. The white girl tells her friend never to consent. The man nods his head and the men begin. They put her on the floor and spread her legs wide, and a man holds each leg apart. Her hands are tied to posts in the floor. A man touches her cunt and starts to play with it. Another sucks her nipples. They start to finger her; then one after the other, they fuck her. After the last one gets off her, the man who had kidnapped her snaps his fingers and in comes a huge black man. He comes to her and puts a pillow under her ass and looks at her, laughing. His cock is huge—at least nine inches, and he tells her he's going to fuck her until she sees stars. She starts to breathe heavy, and he kisses her mouth and then her breasts. He sucks her nipples and rubs them with his fingers. He pinches them until she starts to moan. He puts two fingers in her cunt, and the girl starts trying to fuck his fingers. He puts his mouth to her open pussy lips and kisses the lips. He sucks them and her clit. Then he thrusts his tongue in her wet pussy. She's wild with passion. Then he moves between her legs and guides his erect and throbbing cock into her hot and wet cunt. She's so wet, he almost slips out. He thrusts a couple of times, and she comes one, two, three times. He hasn't come, but he takes his wet penis out of her hungry pussy, and she starts crying for him to fuck her more. He laughs, and the men move to her and wash her out and give her a douche. The black man tells them to untie her. They comply, and she rises to embrace him, but the men put her on her stomach and spread her legs wide apart. The black man starts to finger her pussy, and she starts moaning and getting wet. The black man fucks her pussy, and she cries out. He spanks her ass and spreads her ass and starts fingering her asshole. She begs him to fuck her in the ass, and he laughs. He moves down and starts licking and sucking her wet snatch. She has another big orgasm. The man who kidnapped the two girls now tells the blonde she belongs to the black man. She kisses his feet in gratitude. The kidnapper now looks at the pretty black girl and asks her if she will forgive him, that he loves her and would be forever grateful if she would stay with him. She agrees. The End.

The next fantasy I was too embarrassed to tell my fiancé. He knows I like gay guys, but he doesn't know that they are to me the focal point of the majority of my sexual fantasies. Sometimes when we're making love, I think it would be great if he would have a scene with another great-looking guy, and I could watch and touch them.

Fantasy 2: This fantastic-looking kid, about seventeen, is walking on the beach looking for a spot to sunbathe in the nude. He's wearing a short kimono and comes to a stretch of beach where he spreads his towel down and removes his kimono and, lying down, falls off in a light sleep. Two guys are coming down the beach and spot him. The kid doesn't hear them coming, but feeling their presence, he opens his eyes, and they're standing over him running their eyes up and down his body. He's quite embarrassed, but the guys put him at ease and introduce themselves. They ask him if he'd like them to put suntan oil on his body. He says okay. They take some oil and, rubbing it into their hands, tell him he's got a great body. They start, slowly and sensually, and when they reach his stomach, he becomes erect. They very gently move him on his side. One of the guys moves to his erect cock and takes it in his mouth. The other first puts his finger in his ass, and the boy starts to writhe. He puts oil on his cock and enters him. The boy starts to protest that he's hurting him, but the man enters him slowly and starts to fuck him, pumping hard and fast. The boy meets his thrusts and comes in the other guy's mouth as the guy in back shoots his hot juice in his tight asshole.

Vi

My most delicious fantasy is centered around a motorcycle ride. I have come to an old boyfriend's house for a rare long weekend together—since we now live so far apart. Although he doesn't own his own motorcycle, he has borrowed one from a friend for us to take on a romantic cheese-and-wine picnic. We rise early Sunday morning to avoid any traffic, and the fall air is crisp and clear as we roar away, the wind blowing my hair onto my neck. I have driven the bike briefly the day before, and when we reach the lush countryside, I yell over the roar that I want to take the controls. Because the cycle is not his and is such a powerful machine, I really have to coax him (as only I know how!) until he finally relents.

When we switch positions, we both decide to remove our denim jackets. I feel the smooth rush of power available to me whenever I ask for it, and as we reach the crest of a short hill, I accelerate just enough to raise both of us slightly from the seat. As my tight pants stretch across my crotch, I become aware of the engine's throbbing heat against it, as if I were riding a huge flying cock.

Quickly, my neck flushes, and I realize how my nipples are erect and aching. The pulsating warmth has crept over me until it is released in a sweltering burst.

Slowing slightly, I deftly reach back my hand and guide his to cup my breast. Quickly, his free hand undoes my bra, and his warm palms caress me. As I bend back to hear what he says, he tongues my ear so that I swerve the bike slightly. Then he takes the controls and drives the machine through a small culvert and into a secluded pine forest where the sun sifts through the swaying branches.

Before he can get to me, I undo his pants and kiss his ferocious cock on all sides, on top, before sucking it into my mouth. He falls back onto the pine needles with a groan as I slip his warm meat into my mouth and then completely encircle it with my tongue, which I love to do. We undress one another completely as my mouth continues to play with his dick.

Tenderly, he pushes me onto my back as he goes down on my cunt hairs, already wet. I stare up passion drunk at the treetopped sky until our frenzy forces me to shut my eyes. He tongue-teases me all over my body until our mouths meet, and then slowly, ever so slowly, he puts his fire up my cunt. It seems to continue going in forever deeper, deeper. I move side to side as he thrusts away, matching his rhythm. Suddenly, his juices go straight in me, just as I am washed away in my ocean of orgasm. At this point, my real orgasm with my real lover coincides with my fantasy orgasm!

CHAPTER EIGHT

DREAMS COME TRUE

☐ One of the great misconceptions about sexual fantasy is that they are suppressed wishes. The first shock is to accept the fact that not only do women have feelings of lust, too, but that they like to use their imagination to heighten these erotic desires. But once past the notion that all women are "ladies"—meaning sexless—there is a great, fuzzy-minded leap forward: if women enjoy thinking about these bizarre sexual events, *it must mean that they really want to do them!*

The notion that a woman may be thinking these highly charged thoughts puts many a man off. Anxious ideas of competition are aroused; how can he match the prodigious feats of the athletic Adonis in her mind? It is much easier for him to feel she doesn't merely get a kick out of thinking about these things. He decides she really wants to *do* them, probably has done them in the past with other men. In this way, she has been safely put into the category of "freaky," "strange," and "different." There's nothing wrong with *his* sexuality; she's the crazy one.

"What does your husband think about your wanting to be fucked by two strange guys at a football game?" men leer at me, having read the opening pages of *My Secret Garden*, in which I talk about one of my former favorite fantasies—which took place in a football stadium. Another guy nudges me: "Hey, I have two tickets for the Baltimore Colts' game. How about it?"

When you put your name to a book of sexual fantasies, you automatically come to be thought of as a woman who wants to act them all out. Nothing could be farther from the truth. I have no more real desire to be fucked at a Baltimore Colt-Minnesota Viking football game by two unknown men, than I do to be fucked by anyone, anywhere, than in the usual place(s) my husband and I do it. If my fantasies sound outrageous to many people, it is probably because of the conventional manner in which I was brought up. Had I been raised in a whorehouse, perhaps the images that would arouse me to tremendous passion would be scenes of a handsome knight in white armor—looking a bit like Robert Redford—who would make love to me in a house designed by *Bride* magazine, while an organ played "Oh, Promise Me."

My childhood and adolescence were studded thick and fast with sexual rules very much like yours. It left me with an imagination that gets off on the wildest, most forbidden sexual imagery—all of which has little to do with how I live in the real world. I relish the totally unacceptable in my fantsies. I love my life the way it is. If I try to understand without judging the extraordinary diversity of sexual experience available to us, it does not necessarily mean I contain within myself all the points of view put forward by the several hundred women whose fantasies I published. And yet I have appeared on various radio and television talk shows where the hosts and other guests have actually become angry when I wouldn't bend the entire meaning of my understanding of sexual fantasy to conform with their ideas: namely, that sexual freedom, greater sexual pleasure, must mean having all our sexual dreams come true. "What, you only think these ideas and don't act them out? Isn't that hypocritical, copping out?"

My answer is, No. As you will see from this chapter, there are many people who have found sheer bliss in joining with their partners in acting out their sexual fantasies as if they were dramatic scripts for two (or more) players. That's terrific, for them. But most of the women who have written me are far from wanting to put their fantasies into fact. They go out of their way to say it to me in so many words: "I love to imagine these things but I have no desire to really do them." If that is where they draw the line, they have every right to. They are no less "daring" or adventurous than the people who act out their fantasies. Just different.

Probably the greatest sexual and social gain we could reach will be when we become liberated enough to allow each one his or her own sexual inclination. We are still so insecure in our own sexual tastes and identities that people with other ideas make us anxious. We hold to whatever norm has been okayed in the latest book and is most widely held to be right by our neighbors. Anyone who dares to operate an inch outside of this accepted area is ostracized as odd, perverted.

The people in this chapter fall outside neat categories. Not only do they have sexual desires that other people never talk about, but they have mentioned them to their lovers and/or husbands. They've even gone wilder than that: they've proceeded to act out what was on their minds. Whether or not they found pleasure in following their erotic scenarios is their business; what is more important to our discussion is understanding that they felt free enough, accepting enough with each other, to acknowledge that's where their desires lay, and to act upon them.

I think that for every person who has written to me about the joys of performing their sexual dreams in reality, there have been three or four who knew in advance that it wouldn't work, or who tried it and were disappointed. Whether or not you decide to try yours out in reality is up to you, but I would argue to the death with anyone who says that unless you do you are only going halfway. What turns them on is their business; what turns you on is yours. The U.S. Commission's Report on Obscenity and Pornography showed that both men and women responded with far more excitement when they were asked to imagine something erotic than when they actually saw it.

But if the majority of people I have heard from say

it is more exciting (or less threatening) to keep their sexual fantasies only in the mind, it is still not the whole sexual truth: to be honest about sex, you can't merely count heads and pronounce judgment democratically. Individual differences must be considered and accepted to be as valid as the tastes of the majority. The people who have put their erotic fantasies into practice are neither braver than you or I nor more or less daring or self-destructive. They have simply found that a whole new dimension is added to their lives when they act out their fantasies. They have found their own path to a more vivid life. Who's against that?

If you are truly liberated, you must be able to accept that someone who does or thinks something abhorrent to you is not a sexual threat. You have to get over thinking that just because someone else does something that you must do it too (this unconscious feeling that someone else's action is a dare to us to do it, drives us to put up a wall of dislike and disgust between them and us). Next, accept the reality that there are sexual events going on, fantasies being acted out, that you would never imagine. Some of the nicest people you know may be doing the most extraordinary things behind their closed doors. "It may be just because two people get off on the most outrageous, antisocial conduct when they are alone together in their bedroom," a psychiatrist friend said to me recently, "that they very often can be the nicest, easiest, and most socially delightful people to be around at other times. They have expressed all their negative drives with each other, and so are ready to turn their nicest face forward when they meet you." This is no more dishonest than to say you're not hungry after you've eaten.

In psychoanalytic parlance, there is a technical phrase called, "acting out," and while I have used this phrase myself often enough in this chapter, I wish to be clear that I am using it in the common, everyday sense, and not technically, as the doctors do. To them, *acting out* means that a person performs certain actions, usually self-destructive or self-defeating, for reasons she does not understand. Because the basic motivation is repressed to a level below consciousness, the actress is not aware that her behavior is an expression of an *unconscious* fantasy, nor does she have a significant area of choice in the matter: her neurosis compels her through a hidden logic of its own, to find only married, unavailable men attractive, or to behave in such a manner that she is always the victim, getting fired, being taken advantage of, etc., etc.

The women in this chapter, on the contrary, are very much aware of their fantasies: the choice of bringing them into reality or not is entirely their own. Therefore, even though we may call these actions *acting out*, it should be remembered that the way I intend to use the phrase entails very conscious decision. Above all, while the fantasies they decide to live out may at times entail a degree of psychic or physical pain, that is not what they are all about. These women are not about self-defeat and martyrdom—their true goal in acting out their fantasies is the greatest possible pleasure. Carolyn writes that acting out her fantasies brought her so much fulfillment, she has introduced them to her new lover. "He loves it!" she writes ecstatically. "It's a totally new space for him to be in. . . . I don't think I've been in a constant state of turn-on like this, ever. Can't wait until he gets back to act out some more of this lovely state of being."

". . . *this lovely state of being.*" I like Carolyn's phrase. Finding our way to it is the essence of life, but there are no guaranteed roadmaps. It is a place of the spirit, of course, but lovers have always known that it can be reached by physical, sexual means. "The road of excess leads to the palace of wisdom," said William Blake.

Carolyn has found her way; other women in this section have found theirs. □

Carolyn

Okay. Just finished your book and wished with all my being that I didn't have to wait two weeks to share the incredible turn-on I feel from reading it. Masturbation at this level is a "reliever" of sorts, but just doesn't work totally.

Seems to me that what prevents most people from copping to their fantasies to the other person is your basic all-American fear of taking a risk. We're all scared of being thought of as crazies, perverts, or whatever.

I remember the first man who tuned into my fantasies before I even knew I had them. We were both extremely stoned and making foreplay. Suddenly, he stopped doing what he was doing and took a little velvet rope out of his pocket. Without a word, he began to tie my wrists to the bedposts. I could feel that within the little red velvet rope there was a thin, steel chain, so that while the red velvet protected my skin, inside the velvet rope there was this hard, cruel chain that I could never break. I have never been so turned on so fast in all my life. At first, I was afraid that he wasn't going to do what I thought (wanted) he was going to do. Then I was afraid he wouldn't complete the *whole* act to my satisfaction. But he did—taking more velvet chains from a hard-leather executive-type briefcase that he always carried with him, but I had never seen him open before. He slowly tied me in a spread-eagle fashion to the four bedposts, with my arms pulled up and back of my head, my legs spread wide apart and held that way by the chains. He never spoke to me while he did this. He moved like someone in one of my dreams, knowing instinctively what I seemed to want, but never asking me if he was right or wrong about how much I wanted it. He *knew*, and just proceeded with it, crooning to himself all the while, never saying a word, just this intent, bemused, almost gurgling kind of half-humming, half-chuckling. At the end, I could not move a muscle. I was totally in his hands, totally open to whatever he wanted to do to me. I can never remember feeling so incredibly tingly in my whole life. He didn't even have to come near me to get me aroused. All the while I was lying there, I could see that he was looking at me. Really looking. He kept putting his head between my legs, examining the lips of my cunt, taking the flesh delicately in his fingers to hold them open so that he could look in more deeply. But he never went further. As a matter of fact, just leaving me tied up there and leaving the room as if nothing unusual was happening at all was an even greater turn-on. The one feeling I can recall at that moment was one of enormous relief. All these fantasies I could never cop to having were actually being realized by me, and by someone who had the incredible sensitivity to know what I wanted. In this case, *he* was the one who had taken the risk, and for that, I'll forever love him, even though the affair is gone.

My fantasies range along the general line of tie-me-down-spread-eagled-and-do-what-you-or-your-friends-will-with-me (as long as it doesn't hurt). I adore being victimized in a nonthreatening way. Even though, so much of this kind of fantasy does depend on trust of the other person. Trust that he won't slit you from your guggle to your zatch while you're lying there stark naked on the bed, unable to move. The possibility of this happening (remote, one hopes) makes it even more exciting.

I am currently dating a man, much older than I, who's a superlover. But "straight." So, for the first time in my life, I took the risk and turned *him* on to what turned me on. He loves it! It's a totally new space for him to be in, and it's kid-in-the-candy-store time for him (and God knows, for me). I get long letters from him communicating how excited he is with his new state of being. Hear, hear!

Thank you a lot. I don't think I've been in a constant state of turn-on like this ever. Can't wait until he gets back to act out some more of this lovely state of being. If you ever write Volume II, I probably won't be able to get off my bed for the next year!

P.S. I am single and twenty-eight years old.

May

I read your book, and just couldn't resist a chance to tell someone. I'm seventeen, and eight months pregnant and single. I am a very liberated person, sexually and likewise. Sometimes I wonder if I'm perverted or not; I guess I just love sex and always have. I've been having sex (intercourse) for two years now, and have really been the route. I mean I truly feel quite experienced for my age. My first time in bed was with a forty-two-year-old man, or should I say, my girl friend's father. Maybe it sounds pretty lewd, but to this day just the excitement of thinking about anyone finding out about us has an unbelievable effect. We had intercourse several times. One exceptional time was when I stayed at their house for a small slumber party, and when he thought everyone was asleep, he came and got me, and we fucked away in a reclining chair in the living room; well, to add to this, his daughter walked through, but to this day I still wonder how much she really saw. Isn't that a thrill?

I also have this fantasy about large penises. I've always enjoyed very large, filling penises; they seem to excite me the most. I've had the fantasy about being laid by a horse many times, since they are so large, but I don't think it would be possible to live out, but if I had a chance, believe me, I'd jump for it. The most filling fuck ever.

When I was younger, it was my dog that excited me. This was when I was a virgin. I have fucked my dog (German shepherd) many times though. I always wanted a man's penis but was chicken, so I laid the dog. I would lay him on his back on the floor and push the sheath of his penis all the way down, so his penis was just loose, and he would suddenly become so hard and growing that the skin couldn't move back up. He would even start into motion before I was on him. I would squat over him holding that delicious penis straight up, and then I'd come down on him, and, man, that dog could go like hell, sometimes as long as a half an hour, which is long for a dog. He could come and come . . . so would I, ummmm. . . . This I haven't done since I've had intercourse with men, but just thinking about it now makes me wish the dog was around, but someone stole him. I even thought of giving him fellatio, but couldn't.

I have a friend who I am spiritually very close to. I had had fantasies of making deep love to her. One night, she wanted me to meet her lover. She also told me how large he was, which just heightened my curiosity, but I had no intentions of going to bed with him, for I would have felt too guilty. We arrived at his apartment, where there were a few people already there. It was just a social thing at first, sitting around talking and getting high. Well, the conversation somehow came to massages, and I mentioned that I was good at back massages and joint-cracking. This guy said he was too and offered to give me a back massage. I said sure, 'cause I love them. This went on for a while, with me lying facedown on the floor with him sitting on my rear. Next thing I knew, everyone else was too, but they were all in their underwear; then my clothes were being removed, and I just let it happen. By this time, I was getting excited almost to the point of climax, for this guy was sitting on me in his underwear, and I could feel that bulge growing larger and ever warmer and harder. He then tells me to turn over, and he'd give me a front massage, and I thought okay. buddy, I'll play your game and beat you at it too. As my clothes had been removed, I was lying breasts up. looking him right in the face while he sat on my pubic area. He's massaging my stomach and breasts and sending tingles all through my body as I can now see the enormous bulge in his shorts. I am then led into the bedroom and gently laid on the bed while he goes down between my thighs headfirst to further stimulate me with that probing tongue going ever deeper. (My girl friend is sitting beside the bed with that Mother Earth smile, telling me she was just sharing with me what she had found so fulfilling). I was on fire wanting him to enter me, but he teased, further drinking me till I thought I was dry. When he did enter me, I was so alive and eager just begging for more that I came time and time again, while he remarked how good I was in bed, and then it was all over, and we left. This was the most exciting time I ever had, not just because he was so big and good, but the thought of this girl actually sharing this with me. I fantasize about it often now. I loved it. Well, that's enough, my hand's tired, and this is getting a bit long.

Chessie

My fiancé and I both read *My Secret Garden*. We enjoyed it immensely. I'd like to give you some background before I tell my fantasies. I'm nineteen and engaged to be married later this month. I lost my virginity at fourteen, but never masturbated or had many fantasies until I met Lewis. He and I share our fantasies, and there are several that we have acted out or want to act out.

My most frequent (and Lewis' favorite) is that I am at our new home, and a girl that I work with comes over. She is very thin but nicely proportioned. We talk and eventually the conversation comes to sex (which she and I often talk about in reality). We end up sitting there masturbating, which leads into touching each other. We go to the bedroom and touch and kiss. I imagine that she licks and nibbles my breasts (which are large) and eats me. Then I eat her and lick her everywhere. While we are still engrossed, with my mouth against her cunt, Lewis walks in, sheds his clothing, and joins us until we are all exhausted.

There are some variations: other girls that we know; same girl, but her husband walks in too, and there is a quartet, etc. Lewis and I would really above all like to get into a threesome.

Another fantasy goes something like this: I am at a party with Lewis. As we are sitting there, I tell him that I forgot to put on my panties. I am wearing a short dress, but it is not quite short enough to allow him to see anything. All through the party, he is going mad by knowing how I look under that dress. When we get home, I sit down and begin masturbating in front of him. I lift my skirt periodically so that he can see me fondling my cunt and flicking my clit. But when he wants to touch me, I refuse. I do a striptease, again without letting him touch me. Finally, he becomes so hard and so turned on that he tears off my clothes and tries to grab me by the cunt. But I dodge him and make him watch me. I let him lick my fingers; they are running with my juices, but he is not allowed to touch me. He goes mad and tells me that if I don't let him touch me I will be put over his knee. But I still don't give in. He finally catches me and spanks me. Then he bites my breasts (lightly—I'm not hard-core S&M), and puts his cock against my lips. For a moment, I struggle (playfully), and then take his gorgeous cock into my mouth as though it would save my life. Then he goes down on me and eats me until I am in sheer ecstasy. Then he makes me beg for his cock. He teases and tempts me—turning the tables on me—until I am almost crying for him. Then he puts his cock against my cunt and ever so slowly goes deeper. Then he pulls almost all the way out, but just when I think he's going away entirely, he suddenly thrusts deep into me, and we fuck and fuck and fuck, and it is glorious!!!!

We often (in reality) bond one another. The free one teases the bonded one, then touches and kisses and caresses till we are both frantic with longing. Then the free one unties the other, and we fuck away. My favorite thing to do when Lewis is tied is to squat above his mouth, then raise again, just before he has time to lick me. Then, after I masturbate a little, very close to his face, I come down on his mouth. We are very, very happy in our sexual life, and we very much enjoy our fantasies.

Thank you for listening.

P.S. Although I am not interested in making it with an animal, I thought you might be interested in knowing that reading your chapter called "The Zoo" *did* turn me on!

☐ While the women whose fantasies appeared immediately above found that acting out their sexual fantasies were unalloyed bliss, this is not always the case. In translating images from our mind into actual practice, a kind of one-way street opens before us. If something we imagine turns out to distress us, we can always shrug it off. "Oh, well—it was only a passing thought." But once you have put something into action, you can no longer dismiss the reality of it, nor forget the memory if the experience turned out to be unpleasant after all.

The first rule I would suggest if you want to act out one of your fantasies is to be sure you know your lover well and that there is a strong bond of affection between you. Above all, it is important that you have some intuitive feeling that he is doing it just for the kick of it—as you are—and not to express some deeper layer of sexual distortion or rage within himself. If there is a kind of disgust or anger mingled with his excitement—or if he can only go through with the idea of acting out a fantasy when high or drunk—look out. There may well be a postcoital period on his part, not only of sadness, desperation, and regret but also of real fury. His motives for acting out were ambivalent, and not totally about fun. He will try to displace some of his self-contempt upon you.

Rose Ann tells us that she once fell in love "with a rather sadistic woman-hater." While he was excited by acting out spanking fantasies with her, "the more we got into this, the more I loved him . . . and the more he lost respect for me." Fortunately, as we see in her letter, this did not end in crippling her self-esteem. Her basic health and self-acceptance seem to have won out in the end.

What I find interesting about Nessie's approach to acting out her fantasies of "deference and obedience," is that while it turned out that both she and her husband had secretly harbored these desires, they had never mentioned them to each other—each partner in the marriage thought only she/he liked these things. Another example of the deadly silence that rules most bedrooms, killing our desires by suffocating our favorite dreams.

It was only after she had read *My Secret Garden* and had encouraged her husband to read it, that Nessie decided that since other women liked these pleasures, too, she must not be unique. She found "the nerve to tell him [her husband] about my special fantasy and asked him to act it out."

Her agreed, and they began by taking one tentative step. He slapped her. Then they had another talk, in which each one told the other how they felt about it. They both liked it, and Nessie suggested going the next step.

I heartily endorse this experimental, step-by-step approach, especially the effort to try to talk it all through in advance, so that neither one develops new or frightening ideas that the other is not ready for. Once you're into these scenes, the emotions aroused can go right to the head more fiercely than a rush of amyl nitrate—limits must be set up front, especially if you're flirting with the emotions entailed in S&M scenes. What must be agreed in advance is that either partner has the right to say *stop* at any point, and no reason has to be given except that the pain of the experience has begun to outweigh the pleasure. If this is understood in advance, the other partner is not so likely to get her/his feelings hurt, or feel rejected.

"At first," Nessie writes, after they had agreed to go to the next step, "I was nervous that the whole thing was going to be a disappointment, but after he hit me just once, I knew there was no danger of that. It was fantastic."

One woman's pain is another woman's heaven.

Lizzy's letter may not strike you at first as a fantasy at all—until you remember that the entire idea that Lizzy engage in "lesbian sex" with Ethel was the erotic fancy of Lizzy's husband. Before her first date with Ethel, he eagerly entered into a little foreplay with his wife "until I began to lubricate. Then he said, 'Now you're Ethel's,' kissed me and left." In the end, Bill's fantasy has been much more completely acted out than perhaps even he dreamed; it has become what sounds like an extraordinarily open and joyous way of life for all three people.

An interesting, if minor, note to Lizzy's letter is that while she tells us how ecstatically happy she is when in bed with either one of her two beloved partners (and I for one find her very convincing), she nevertheless remains true to the basic theme of fantasy: when she is in the arms of one lover, she closes her eyes and fantasizes that she is with the other. □

Rose Ann

Thank you for your book. How needed it was. I'm glad to have the opportunity to give you some of my experiences. I hope they're interesting.

I'm twenty-three, single, college grad, working as a secretary, gong to grad school for psych in the fall. I've had at least twenty-five sexual relationships with men, half that number with women. I really like both, although it is easier to be passive with men, and as you will see from my fantasies, this is pretty much where it's at for me.

At age four, my six-year-old girl friend and I would play "Witchdoctor." This consisted, from what I recall, of her bending me over a box in my mother's closet, pulling down my pants, and inserting her finger into my ass. I really used to get off on this (age four?), and the Witchdoctor theme has persisted until now (with hundreds of variations, of course), until now it is almost impossible for me to climax without a form of this fantasy. Since reading your book, I have discovered that it works to think of the simple act of fucking, or of a woman (in whom I may be interested at the moment) eating me. I never thought these kinds of simple thoughts could turn me on enough (too normal) to help me come. But thanks to you, my "fantasy bank" has suddenly doubled in value.

About me: I masturbate all the time. Most every day (whether I'm having a relationship or not). Lot of times, if I stay home from work one day or on a Saturday when I don't feel like going out, I can lie in bed all day and come again and again and feel like I haven't wasted my day at all. Last night, I came nine times before going to sleep. Anyway . . . let's get into my fantasy.

The main elements are my passivity at the hands of this doctor or whoever (it's never a rapist). (Once after going through customs on the way back from Mexico, and being told by the customs guy that "We can strip you, you know, if we think you've got dope on you," I did a whole new fantasy on being examined and searched by these sex-hungry customs men and women. They're never rough, always very calm and methodical, even when they're making me suck them off.)

In the main fantasy that I've had since childhood, a a mad doctor has somehow abducted me. I am in his laboratory (he is in a white lab coat—faceless, of course). He has me strapped down to an unusual examining table. Sometimes the table branches out into a "v" at the bottom, so my legs can be securely strapped wide open to each arm of the "v," and the doctor has easy access to my genitals. There are little metal caps which are placed over my nipples. Wide metal circular bands which fit around my breasts, which hold them up straight into the air. Sometimes hot needles are inserted into my nipples (I have done this myself sometimes and have been very stimulated if I don't hurt myself too much). I am usually blindfolded and gagged, or my mouth is propped open. The main apparatus has, as its base, a huge black ceiling-height metal thing (like the X-ray business in a dentist's office). . . . From this, on the end of a spring kind of thing, comes the actual device that will penetrate my genital/anal areas. This latter, when inside me, will buzz, vibrate, be electrically shocking in some way. The device for my lower regions is three-pronged. From the center of it protrudes a phallic thing, shiny metal, smooth, and huge. This is inserted into my vagina. (By the way, the "doctor" always uses words that are very clinical: "vagina," "anus," etc., never "cunt" or "ass." Sometimes there is an assistant there whom the doctor orders about, "Insert the anal device," "Hold her down," "Strap her arms securely," "Spread her wider," etc. Hearing these words is very important. I say nothing, except an occasional, "Oh, no, please don't." But the doctor is constantly talking, if not to his assistant, then to me: "Just relax," "Hold still," "That's good," "Don't move," "Just lie still," etc. He is always extremely calm and self-possessed, never becoming excited or anything.) The second "arm" of the device is a smaller version of the vaginal device, it is for my anus. The third section looks like a miniature floor waxer. It is a little round rubber thing (something like a washer for a faucet) which is on the end of a short metal rod. This is positioned on my clitoris. It will, when activated, spin 'round and 'round like a floor waxer, "waxing" my clit to climax.

Although certain things vary, this is basically the one fantasy to which I've climaxed for like eight years. I also get off on thinking of being gently, but forceably bent over a table or something and being penetrated by a finger or a cock or a vibrator in my ass. Actually, having hemorrhoids, I can't do anything like this, unfortunately.

I have had the good fortune to have almost acted out my doctor fantasy. This doctor is not your typical professional, as you will see. Coming back from Florida one summer with a bad case of scabies, I went to this guy on the recommendation of a friend. Going late in the afternoon (after work), his office was empty except for me and his nurse, and she was off someplace far from the examining room. Instead of giving me a gown or something or calling in the nurse (as I believe doctors are required to do by law), he just told me to "take down my pants and bend over the table" (the scabies were on my ass). Needless to say, I immediately became so aroused I thought I was going to faint. But all he did was poke around at the scabies and give me a prescription and a date for a second exam. Well, by the time the day for the second exam came around, I was determined (encouraged by his unorthodox methods) to have something happen. Just what that would be, I wasn't sure, but I was determined. So, after a repeat of the first performance, I began my spiel. "Dr. So-and-so, I don't really know who else to tell this to, or where to turn for help. I'm twenty-two years old and have never had an orgasm. I don't even know what it feels like. What should I do?" I went on and on and on with this oh-so-sincere look and tone of voice. He began his answer by telling me what to tell my boyfriend to do. I countered by saying that I had told my boyfriend things, and that nothing worked. I wouldn't even know what an orgasm was if I fell over one, etc. etc. That's when he told his nurse to go home (it was about 6 P.M.), and I knew I had it in the bag. His next line almost made me laugh out loud with elation. He said, "Have I given you a pelvic? Maybe there is something wrong with you physically. Take off your clothes, and get up on the table." No gown, nothing. Just me COMPLETELY NUDE climbing up on the table. I was so excited I didn't know if I could keep from passing out. Well, the good doctor, surgical glove well lubricated with surgical goo, went straight, and I mean straight, for my clit. His "How does that feel? Tell me. Tell me" bullshit was ruining it, though, and I had to tell him to shut up. Anyway, I came, but was surprised to find that I still had to fantasize that I was bound and tied up before I could make it. Afterward, he wanted to fuck me, but he was actually an ugly little man, and I very hastily thanked him and split. Frankly, it was pretty dreamlike. I couldn't believe I had had the nerve to do it, or that this fantasy had actually come true. But, also frankly, the fantasy is much more satisfying and exciting than that experience was.

Another "fantasy-come-true" happened with a rather

sadistic woman-hater that I was falling madly in love with. He got off first on spanking me. Gradually, we progressed to his tying me down to the bed and whipping the shit out of me with his belt till my breasts, thighs, and ass were bruised for days. I didn't get off on the pain per se, but on the psych of the thing, especially when he would kiss and caress and pity the wounds he had just inflicted. The whippings themselves didn't make me come. I would usually have to masturbate while he was whipping and fucking me (from behind), but if I did concentrate on what was actually going on, it helped to get me off. The mercy trip was the crucial thing here, I think. His loving those parts of my body that he'd just finished wounding. (*Story of O?*) Anyway, the more we got into this, the more I loved him and felt possessed and owned by him, and the more he lost respect for me, and there went that relationship. He wound up calling me a sicky, and telling me how bad I was for him and all. For a while, this made me feel really sick and perverted, but I now realize, at least, that it takes two to make a sick relationship, and besides, what the fuck? How can you say something that is "you" is sick or normal? If it makes up what is in totality "you," it is as unique and unlabelable as is each person walking around this earth. So, that guy's hang-ups, as far as I'm concerned, are his own.

When the movie *The Devils* came out, a whole new fantasy world opened to me. I don't know if you're familiar with it. The "nun-possessed-by-sexual-demons-that-must-be-exorcised-through-sexual-means" type of thing. Vanessa Redgrave, the nun in question, had to go through the most delicious forced tortures (having her breasts bound with barbed wire, etc.) It turned me on so I had to leave in the middle to go home and masturbate. The rape scene from *Rosemary's Baby* did the same. At age seven or eight I saw a television flick about these Martians that landed and were taking over earth by nabbing the town's most prominent folks and drilling these little computerized control devices into the backs of their necks. Watching that movie, I can remember feeling my cunt throbbing like the dickens for the first time. Watching this beautiful, utterly passive woman, her neck bent forward, and this drill beginning to enter her neck . . . wow. I remember my mother came in and wanted to tell me something just as this was happening, and I threw something at her. I was so wrapped up and throbbing and angry that she'd disturbed me. Of course, she thought I was just into the flick. She didn't know why, I'm sure, but she didn't talk to me for days 'cause of my throwing something at her.

I usually don't fantasize about women while I'm masturbating or fucking, except rarely, when I've met a woman I'd really like to sleep with and don't know if she's up for it or not. Since reading your book, however, I've found that I can fantasize about a (prospective) female lover eating my cunt deliciously. I'll wind up calling her name and coming like a bitch.

Anyway, best of luck. What you're doing is really dynamite.

Nessie

I have just finished reading *My Secret Garden,* and I thought I would write this as a kind of "thank you."

I bought your book for myself, and that's why I was quite surprised when my husband—who never reads anything—seemed interested in it. It was that that finally gave me the nerve to tell him about my special fantasy and ask him to act it out.

Ever since I was a little girl, I have been turned on by the idea of getting spanked. My parents never did so I don't know how it happened to appeal to me—but it did. As I got older and knew more about sex, my horizons broadened a bit, and I enjoyed the thought of being beaten with a belt.

My whole personality is geared toward male domination—I hate guys who let women walk all over them. Taking this into consideration, my husband is the perfect partner for me, the kind who treats a girl fantastic in return for a little deference and obedience.

But to get back to the subject, sometimes when we were fucking, I'd ask him to slap me, and he always would, although he seemed a little resistant.

The night after we had been reading your book, I got him started slapping me while he fucked me, and after it was over, I thought "what the hell," he knows that other women like weird things, so I'll ask him. I said, "Do you like hitting me?" and he said, "Yes." I asked him if he'd ever thought of trying it with something else. "Like what?" he asked me, and I said, "Like a belt."

He seemed to like the idea, but we were both a little unsure how to get started. I suggested we start with a spanking to sort of warm up. He took me across his knee and slapped my buttocks about ten times; then we got into a foreplay thing, with him kissing me very deeply and fingering my cunt.

I had smoked a joint before all this and that, plus the anticipation of what was going to happen, had me more turned on than I can ever remember being. He asked me if I was ready, and when I said I was (was I ever!) he undressed me and told me to turn over on my stomach.

At first, I was nervous that the whole thing would be a disappointment, but after he hit me just once, I knew there was no danger of that. It was fantastic! It hurt (although not terribly), but I wanted it to go on forever: I can't really describe the feeling, except that I loved feeling helpless, and that he was so much stronger, more dominant than I was.

We talked about it afterward, and it turned out that he'd always dug that type of thing too, but was afraid to broach the subject to me. Thank goodness your book gave me the nerve to bring it up, or I might never have known.

So I guess that while some fantasies aren't ideal when turned into reality, this one sure was. And it's all because of you, really, so thanks a lot.

Kellie

I have just finished reading *My Secret Garden,* and found it to be one of the most interesting books I've read in ages. I thought I might enjoy sharing my thoughts with you.

I am twenty-three years old, and my husband is twenty-six. We have been married for six years and have two children.

I was surprised that most of the men you talked with were so closed-minded about the existence of women's sexual fantasies. My husband not only admits that they exist but gets very turned on when I share my fantasies with him. Our sexual relationship has always been good, but it gets more exciting all the time, due to our fantasy-sharing.

I suppose my fantasies are typical. My favorite being that I am seduced by an attractive man; sometimes he is someone we know; more often, he is a stranger. I later tell my husband all the details, relating it exactly, word for word, action by action. Telling my husband what has happened to me is probably the most exciting part of the fantasy. My husband insists that he actually wants me to act out this fantasy. He wants to perform cunnilingus on me (which has always been included in our lovemaking) while I tell him what went on with this fantasy man. He wants to hear everything the man does to me, just as I tell him about it in my fantasy. He says just thinking about it makes him climax. I admit that I am seriously considering doing it, but I'm afraid of jeopardizing our relationship. My husband and I are very close to each other, and this is important to me. The interesting thing is that my husband is very jealous and possessive of me, and I'm afraid that if I really did act out this fantasy, that it might not have the desired effect. However, he insists that it would not hurt our relationship, but would add to it, as long as I am completely honest with him.

Another fantasy of ours is making it with a black man.

Yes, my husband would actually like to "go down" on a black cock, with me watching all the action. Even though most men would not admit to being turned on by another man's cock, my husband does and is. He actually had an experience with a black man when he was in the service, and had been drinking quite a bit. He told me everything that happened, and it did not repulse me in any way. In fact, it had quite the opposite effect. It does not make him less of a man in my eyes. I know he is not a true homosexual, as he has proven that through our relationship. But the thought that he enjoys sex so much, that he thinks of pleasing men too, makes his sexuality all the stronger to me. Know what I mean? I really dig his honesty.

Well, I guess I've gone on long enough. I hope that I've been able to add something useful to your studies.

P.S. My husband has read this letter and has approved my sending it to you.

Lizzy

I've just finished a wonderful experience—reading *Secret Garden*—and am taking advantage of your request to send on further experiences.

It was great to know that I'm not alone in fantasizing, or in actually using four-letter words, which I now love. In your sequel, I hope you will pay more sympathetic attention to lesbian relationships, which changed my own life.

For background—I am thirty-eight years of age, married fifteen years to a wonderful man whom I love dearly, and we have three lovely children. My dear husband paid every possible attention to me during our marriage, and made every effort to give me sexual satisfaction. Over the years, he fucked me constantly, entered me from the rear, went down on me, gave me hours of foreplay, all to no avail. No matter what he did, I simply couldn't come. Incidentally, I was a virgin when we married. He tried being gentle, rough, raped me in the middle of the night, and nothing helped. I enjoyed being close to him, and during any sex, I'd start to lubricate, get soaked, and then I'd dry up. By the time he'd come in my cunt, I was just waiting for him to finish.

My husband was frantic to make me come, the darling, but of course he was enjoying me less and less, as he felt very selfish coming when I didn't. Then he brought some magazine featuring male nudes in an effort to arouse me, but they did nothing for me. When those failed, he brought home some girlie magazines, the porno types, featuring lesbian sex acts. I found those exciting, and told him so, so he had me read them, and then he'd go down on me, or fuck me, and while it was more exciting, I still couldn't come.

After some weeks of this, my husband told me that his opinion was that our problem was that what I sub-consciously wanted was sex with a woman, and, as he put it, this might open the dam. When I objected, he reminded me that our own sex acts were getting more and more infrequent, and he admitted to me this was because he preferred to masturbate rather than subject me to the torture of being aroused and then frustrated. So I asked where one would find a woman, and he laughed and said that if I opened my eyes a bit, I'd see that a certain very dear friend of mine was more than casually interested in me.

Well, for several weeks after that, I watched her very carefully each time we had coffee together, or went shopping, etc., and little by little, I became convinced that my husband might just be right. My girl friend, who was also married and several years younger than I was, certainly displayed more interest than I had noticed. I noticed, for one thing, that each time we met, her eyes went over my figure from top to bottom, with special emphasis in the area of my tits, which are a firm 37. Now that I'd been alerted, I noticed also that as we'd have coffee or lunch, her eyes were much more on my chest than on my face, and I concluded that my husband had read the signs correctly. Also, I began to look her over, and found her very sexy-looking. I began to fantasize what it would be like to really make love to her. I practiced, in my mind, and really enjoyed it. Then, little by little, she introduced the subject of sex, and after a while lesbian sex, which she said she practiced and loved. When I asked if this didn't lessen her pleasure with her husband, she said that, quite to the contrary, it added to her marital relations. She (let me call her Ethel) told me her husband knew and fully approved, and had in fact joined her and her girl friend at times, and that these experiences stimulated both of them to better and wilder sex. At one point, she told me outright she was propositioning me, that I was the sexiest-looking female she'd ever seen, and had always wanted to go to bed with me. Incidentally, she was a believer in earthy language, and what she actually said was that she wanted to suck my tits, go down on me. My husband had never used such language with me, but I found myself quite excited when she talked about "fucking, sucking," etc., and I also enjoyed her references to tits, cunts, cocks, pricks, asses, etc.

Briefly, my husband continued to encourage me to try sex with Ethel, with whom I finally made a date to visit at her home one morning when her husband would be at work. My husband, whom I'll call Bill, was delighted for me. In fact, before he left for work that morning, he subjected me to some foreplay, ended by going down on me only until I began to lubricate. Then he said, "Now you're Ethel's," kissed me and left.

I showered, dressed, and drove to Ethel's. When I arrived, she was wearing just a sheer negligee, through which I could quite plainly see her tits, and the vague outline of her cunt. When she saw my reaction, she smiled, kissed me on the lips, her tongue parted my lips and entered my mouth, and she had my juices flowing again. From here on begins the fantasy which I indulge in now whenever my husband goes down on me, fucks me, front or rear, and we have a sixty-nine. When I am particularly desirous of a long fantasy, Bill will go down on me for an hour or more so that I can relive my experiences with Ethel. All these experiences, in the rest of this letter, when we lived together in fantasy, have really made my real sex life beautiful.

After a bit, she led me to the bedroom, where she first removed her negligee. Her naked body did excite me—her tits were smaller than mine, but beautifully shaped, with sexy nipples which were erect. Her body was lovely, and what stimulated me greatly was that her cunt was clean shaven. She was a beautiful sight, and looking at her, I realized how right my husband had been—I found her extremely desirable.

She came to me, kissed me again, placed my hand on her tit, which I must admit felt terrific. I never expected a woman could feel so exciting, which I suppose sounds very naïve. Then she began to undress me. while I continued to fondle her tits, to my own surprise. When my bra came off, she exclaimed over my beautiful tits, caressed them, rubbed the nipples, and sucked them till they came erect. Last off were my panties, whereupon she knelt and kissed my cunt. Then she told me how beautiful I was, that I had the most desirable body in the world, that she wanted me desperately, etc. Between her talking and playing with me, she had me going very nicely, you can be sure. It also served to make me forget that she was female, and she became just someone else who desired me passionately.

She then laid me down on the bed, laid down beside me, and subjected me to a very long period of foreplay. She kissed me from head to toe, turned me over, and did the same to my backside, turned me back, kissed me with her tongue in my mouth for a long period, sucked my nipples, lingered at my thighs, kept telling me how much she wanted me for what seemed like hours, with me getting more and more aroused by the second.

Finally. when I felt that any more would be unbearable, I begged her to get on with whatever she had in mind. With that, she smiled, turned me to lie across their large bed, my hips at the edge. Then she placed two pillows under my head, explaining that half the thrill of getting sucked off was to be able to watch it as well. She then knelt before me, spread my legs, lifted them until my knees were at my chest, and began the most incredible experience of my life. Her tongue ranged my thighs, came up to my cunt, roamed the outer lips, came down and through my inner cunt, circled the clitoris, came down again and circled the inner lips, the inner wall, repeated this innumerable times, came slowly up after I don't know how long, circled the clitoris, flicked across it, sideways, then up and down, then sucked it in between her lips, licked it rapidly now, circled it more rapidly, began to lick me faster and more demandingly, brought me up several times more, till I thought I'd go mad. Finally, she decided to make me come, and now she concentrated on my clitoris, licking it up and down faster and faster. And then it happened! I had expected that I'd soon begin to dry up as usual, but seeing Ethel's loving head between my legs, feeling her magnificent tongue in me, I found my juices flowing more and more; then suddenly, I felt my stomach muscles begin to contract violently. Every feeling was centered in my cunt, my legs went down and closed around Ethel's head, and as she continued to lick me, I felt as if I were exploding, and I began to come. My body convulsed, my hips came up off the bed, and Ethel had all she could do to stay with me. With my first orgasm, my darling Ethel just sucked in on my clitoris; in between, she licked it rapidly, and with each succeeding orgasm she sucked me in, then licked me again, etc. You must understand that each orgasm was a real convulsion, each one forced a shriek from me, as this was the culmination of so many years of frustrated sex. According to Ethel, I had somewhere around twenty orgasms that first time, and I for one can believe it. After my last orgasm, Ethel kept her tongue in my cunt, no movement, just holding it comfortingly against the upper wall and clitoris, ready if any further orgasms occurred. After some five minutes or so, I did have one of those delayed spasms, so she merely licked the clitoris very gently till it was over.

Nancy, she was real good, but so is Bill, and the difference was in having a woman go down on you, seeing a female head between your legs. How right Bill and Ethel both were! As long as I live I will never forget that first climax, and will always be grateful to Ethel.

After I had rested awhile, lying in Ethel's arms, full of gratitude, I put my hand to her tit, which again felt wonderful, kissed her, feeling that I owed her quite a bit, then ran my hand down to her clean cunt, which fascinated me. I had never even thought about going down on a woman, had often thought that the odor or taste must be unpleasant, but with Ethel, it was different, as I didn't give these things a thought. I was so grateful I'd have done anything for her. As I proceeded with foreplay, Ethel said it wasn't necessary for me to reciprocate, that it would be enough for her to masturbate, and her husband would give her anything she required. I'm glad to say I was woman enough to insist, and I followed the type of foreplay she had used on me, although not so long. When I put a finger in her cunt, I found her very wet, which excited me to think I could do this to her. When I got around to using my tongue on her body, I loved sucking her nipples, her thighs, and, rather to my surprise, I found that her cunt not only smelled great but tasted wonderful. It was at that moment that I understood why Bill so enjoyed going down on me.

As an aside, if my typing is a bit erratic, Nancy, I've been masturbating through much of it, because the memory is so intensely exciting that my juices flow like mad when I think about it, let alone write about it. I've come twice so far, once with a finger and once with a dildo, so I can now continue.

Well, I ended that first time by sucking her off in her favorite position—I lay flat on my back, she straddled my head, lowered herself till I could reach her cunt and clitoris easily, and she kept her upper lips spread to give me full access. Also, in this position, she had me feel her tits throughout, rubbing her nipples, fondling her, etc., and right before she was ready to come, she had me put one arm around her, and insert a finger in her ass. She explained that the combination of my finger with the strain of straddling me, made for a more intense climax, and judging from the results, she was right. I just loved sucking her off, and licking her stiff clitoris was out of sight. When I came before, I was somewhat embarrassed that I had shrieked with each spasm, and when Ethel came very violently, I was delighted that she also tended to scream while coming. When I was through with her, I felt like a million, because my first time out, I had enjoyed the greatest of all thrills—making somebody come intensely, most especially a woman, as making a man come is automatic.

Before we finished that first day, Ethel introduced me to a female sixty-nine, which I also loved, and we fucked each other, at the same time, as strange as that may sound. Ethel had what she called a double dildo, eighteen inches long, with an imitation head and balls on each end. Before our first sixty-nine, she and I had mutual foreplay for some time. Then when we were both flowing greatly, she opened a drawer and took out this giant dildo and explained its use to me, asking if I felt like trying it. By then I was ready for anything, so I said fine. So she lay me on my back, inserted about five or six inches in my cunt, had me turn on my side with one leg raised. Then she lay opposite me, put her legs between mine and slowly worked her way into her end of the dildo. With that, she began to pump, told me to do likewise, and we developed a nice rhythm as I do when fucking Bill. It was marvelous! The rubber dildo felt like a man's cock, you could control how much you wanted, and I could watch Ethel fucking away just as I was. I'd never thought such a thing possible, but you live and learn.

Anyhow, we spent six or seven hours together that day, and Ethel made me come I don't know how many times. Before I left her that day, she'd made a woman out of me, that's for sure.

When I got home that day, I was all female. I should mention that, before I left Ethel that day, she was very concerned about my relations with Bill. After she and I had had a great deal of sex, about an hour before we were due to part, she said I must be prepared for Bill. So she gave me about an hour of preliminaries, got me lubricating thoroughly, and then sent me home!

Well, I told Bill all about it that evening, of course, and excited him no end. He was delirious at the thought that I had actually come, and couldn't wait to get to me. While we were at dinner, he kissed me, felt my tits, put his hand under my dress, tongued me, and in spite of all the times I had come with Ethel, he had me flowing again. When I felt his cock, it was hard as could be, and when he fucked me well before dinner was done, for the first time in our married life, I came! Then he went down on me, and I came again. Finally I went down on him, and believe it or not, while I was sucking his cock, I myself came once more! All this I owed to Ethel!

Bill insisted that I continue to see Ethel, which I, of course, was most happy to do, and I've continued to have sex with her since. I keep Bill fully advised of what goes on between Ethel and me, which stimulates him no end. When I came home after my first experience with Ethel, Bill and I had a whole night of sex—he fucked me, went down on me, we had a sixty-nine. I must admit that, after Ethel, Bill looked better to me than ever before, and more important, the first time Bill sucked my cunt, I came beautifully, and even more significant, when he fucked me, I came for him, and this was the greatest gift he could have received!

Since then, Bill has expanded his thinking on sex. With his urging, I still see Ethel several times a week, and I religiously tell Bill everything that goes on between Ethel and me. After each time I have sex with Ethel, sex with Bill is much more exciting and satisfying.

Additionally, Bill has now brought me some new

appliances, as I've also learned to masturbate satisfactorily. He brought me, for instance, a very sophisticated dildo with a rubber bulb, which one fills with warm soapy liquid. When I jerk off with it, which is frequent because Bill travels quite a lot, I use it to fuck myself (it's nine inches long, like Bill), but when I'm ready to come, I just squeeze the bulb, and the warm soapy liquid just like Bill's semen squirts into my cunt, so it's pretty much like having Bill there. More often, though, Ethel is with me and fucks me with the dildo, or sometimes Bill himself does it for me. The point is, Nancy, that either Ethel or Bill can make me come today easily. Bill travels quite a bit, and when Ethel is not available, he telephones me at night and directs me in the use of this great dildo.

Ethel made it possible for Bill to make me come almost at will. Today, he can fuck me and make me come, go down on me, screw me in the ass, and, very strangly, even when I go down on him, I can also come. All of this because I'm thinking of Ethel at all times.,

I must mention that Ethel also introduced me to another marvelous act. At one point, she inserts a dildo deep in me, had me across the bed; then she sits beside me, spreads my cunt's lips, and licks my clitoris while she fucks me with the dildo. Bill does this also, now—very effective!

While I was with Ethel, she suggested to me that my cunt would be much more attractive if I would shave it clean. She said she'd be glad to do the job for me, or Bill could. When I suggested this to Bill, he was thrilled, and that very same night, he stripped me, undressed himself, first used a scissors, then a woman's electric razor, and shaved me clean. When he saw my naked cunt, he went down on me at once, and my cunt had the same effect on Ethel. Both said it was the most beautiful cunt ever, and since then, Bill and Ethel have taken turns shaving me. After each time, I get sucked off, which is great.

Now, Nancy, I come regularly, with almost anything

that's done to me. Bill fucks me, and I come; he goes down on me, and I come; he fucks me in the ass, and I come; he puts a dildo in my cunt and sucks my clitoris, and I come; Ethel goes down on me, and I come; she fucks me with a dildo, and I come; with her or Bill I have a sixty-nine and I come; when I masturbate with a finger or a dildo, I come. (Time out right now for coming with a dildo in my cunt.)

Whether you use any part of this letter or not, Nancy, it's been a great pleasure to write it. More than anything, it's great to be able to use basic language, as men do. Since my experience with Ethel, my husband uses appropriate four-letter words, which thrill me. Where before he used to say, "let's have intercourse," he now says, and I answer in kind, "Let's fuck, dear, or I want to suck your cunt or fuck you with a dildo." In reply I tell him, "Fuck me, Bill, screw me in the ass, suck my cunt, or I want to suck your cock." Ethel uses the same type of language, as I do with her, and she'll phone me, for instance, and say, "Lizzy, darling, let's get together today so I can suck you off, fuck you with a dildo, or let's have a fuck with a double dildo."

Also since Ethel, I've masturbated almost daily, as I find I'm much more sexual than I had thought. When I'm in real need, I'll phone Bill at his office, and he'll instruct me how to masturbate over the phone. If he's alone, he'll also jerk off while we're talking. He'll tell me to arouse myself by feeling my tits and nipples, jerk myself off with a finger, then just how to insert the dildo, fucking me by phone and always making me come.

This is the point of it all, Nancy, which is that for some women such as me what it takes is another woman. For this reason, I urge that, if you are publishing a sequel, a bit more attention be paid to lesbian sex, which has saved me from a life of frustration, and also figures to do the same for many other women. After every session I have with Ethel, Bill is sexier than ever. After a day spent with her, Bill spends most of the night fucking me, going down on me, having sixty-nines, etc. All through sex with him and Ethel, I just keep coming like crazy, and if you ask me who's more effective, I couldn't really say. Now that my cunt is clean-shaven, Bill fucks me and goes down on me more than ever, and he insists that I have sex with Ethel at least a few times a week. As Bill predicted, the dam is broken, and I come almost at will. Also, I don't have to tell you that to be aroused, I don't need the actual experience, just the fantasy of it will do the trick.

So, Nancy, if you do publish a sequel, please stress lesbian sex much more, as there must be thousands of women who are in the position I was. Bill and I were never happier, never had more sex, and I enjoy both of them completely. Bill fucks and sucks me off on the average of ten or twelve times per week, plus at least two days with Ethel. In addition, I masturbate four or five times per week when Bill is home, twice that when he's away.

As a postscript, Ethel is now after me to join her and her husband in a threesome, but I've suggested that she join Bill and me instead. In a foursome, I suppose it would be expected that the two men have sex as well, and this is not for Bill, although Ethel has hinted that her husband might not be averse. We shall see! I'll keep you advised.

Again, Nancy, it's been a great pleasure to be able to write frankly. Sex with women and men is wonderful, and I would like to think that I have helped many other women make up their minds.

P.S. I've masturbated three times during this letter, so whether you use it or not, I've benefited by three great climaxes. Like I said, just thinking or writing about my past experiences, my fantasies, turns me on.

☐ I have chosen the letter that follows to be the last in this book, because it sums up for me all that is best about women's sexuality. Joni acts out her own fantasies, and those of her lover too; she even made a living "for

three months" out of one of them. Her fantasies are as
varied and unexpected as some of the best kinds of sex
itself—cheerful, self-accepting, and even humorous, but
filled with women's unending desire to see sex as a vehicle
for a more abundant life. Joni is serious in her writing,
but never heavy, imaginative to the point of approaching
science fiction, but so filled with the erotic juices of life
that her futuristic machines are never more important
than her lusty women and men.

Joni tells me that her letter contains her "own very
genuine fantasy." The fact that she has put it into skillful
story form does not mean that the emotions are not as
real as those in any other woman's fantasy. All fantasies
are "made up." Joni's are made up by a writer. That's
all. □

Joni

Since childhood, I've wanted to be a dancer—with a
streak of exhibitionistic sexuality involved. There is
something sexually seductive about performing dances.
In earliest puberty (or before—I can't remember exactly)
I daydreamed such old-fashioned things as being a
maiden captured and forced to dance naked for the enjoyment of a sultan or Arabian prince (who no doubt
fell in love with me and married me to make the fantasy
proper and respectable). In adolescence, I admitted to
a secret desire to be a stripper. But to my inhibited and
puritanically raised mind, such an ambition could never
be realized, and so I used to dream of being a movie
star who played the role of a stripper in a film. Talk
about inhibitions! This desire of mine was certainly never
mentioned, let alone fulfilled, after I married a very
puritanical husband (he was a lousy lover, and we were
never good friends, either), but, luckily, I met a man
who uninhibited me (we've been living together for almost
seven years now). His own fantasies centered around
the element of the brazen femme fatale—strippers, women

who pose in provocative stages of dress and undress in men's magazines—so in his presence, hurray! I can live my fantasies and please both of us! When I told him of my secret desire to be an honest-to-God stripper . . . he encouraged me.

I put together an "act." And I performed it to an audience in a topless bar for over three months. The audiences were impressed—they grew larger every week. I was as sexy and seductive as I could possibly be—putting on an act, that is. Something about patterning it, performing over and over, makes it grow stale—a job to be done. It was really marvelous fun, at first, but to keep on creating new acts and dances and props was distracting to my number one Art, that of writing. And the old got boring, and not particularly sexy after a while. I was an actress, performer, creative artist, more than a woman involved in sexual pleasures. I gave it up, but not before I'd enjoyed the sensation of inspiring desire in many men, and pretty well fulfilling—as best as reality can—my secret ambition. I still love to dance seductively. And I've added a dimension to sexual fantasies (my own) I never had before.

In my fantasies now, it is the future, and I have transcended time. Sexual mores have changed. I am a professional exhibitionist-seductress-prostitute. Every night, I do my job, perform my art, and fulfill my sexual needs —all at the same time. In an amphitheater, a large Sex Machine (miracle of science) has been installed. An audience of more than a hundred men pay a big admission price to participate. I am the star. I wear gorgeous clothes—the slinkiest dresses, furs, gloves . . . the most delicate, sexiest underwear. I wear something different every night. I enter the center stage—a sort of glass domed affair with soft spotlights. The men can watch me from little cubicles—one for each man, so he can't be distracted by the others. Electronic waves produce sensations and effects for each man inside his individual room. The glass wall between us is supposed to be one-way, so that they can see me but I don't see them (some are still shy, self-conscious despite the new morality), but actually, I wear contact lenses that enable me to see them all very clearly.

Inside the stage, I begin to seduce them. I slink and recline; dance a little, slowly remove my garments, one by one. I wear a see-through bra and panties, sit on a low couch, one leg drawn up. I roll over, move about. I take off the panties and bra. I dance and move as if I were making love. All the while, I can see each man in his condition of stimulation. A whole sea of erected penises (aroused by my actions) encircle me. I can watch while some of them go into the spasms of orgasm, ejaculating fountains of semen, while they enjoy the exact sensations of having entered my body as I move, as I do . . . and look so desirable. Of course, the Sex Machine works for me, too. Unnown to the men, I can choose any one of them I want, and recreate his exact actions and form in my own body; or I can push any number of buttons (they are hidden under the cushion of the couch) and, in effect, be copulating with ten of them at a time. The sight of me in the midst of orgasm and multiorgasm makes all those who haven't yet climaxed, come, and those who already did, do it again. It's a gigantic orgiastic vision all around me, while I copulate with over a hundred men.

The future holds a promise of much sexual fun for me. Perhaps I am one of the few science-fiction-sexual-fantasists around. Perhaps it's a good way to escape the mundane and the residue of puritanism. The future . . . or life on another planet. What if there were a planet where sexuality had NEVER had an element of forbidden evil? What would it be like? I like to imagine. . . . On this planet (Earth), all pleasures but one are enjoyed without secrecy. We like to eat, and we go to dinner parties and gourmet restaurants. We dance and sing at social functions. We perform and watch the arts. Some of us become gourmets and connoisseurs of various pleasures and arts. What if we could treat sexual pleasure the same way? No, neither brothels nor modern swinger's clubs work the way I have in mind. They lack something—erotic finesse, style. . . . Maybe what I'm thinking of is impossible, because the best sexual designs work between two people who are in tune to each other. It's pretty hard to share and incorporate such personal intimate needs with those very different from yourself. Or is that a false concept created out of my time and place? So far it has been true, but for me in fantasy, one can be a time and space traveler as well as a designer of everything to suit oneself.

I travel to a very far distant time. Life-styles have changed enormously. Sexual needs can be fulfilled in different ways. One can stay home with a lover . . . or go out to charming places. Pleasure Places. A little like a combination of a fine hotel, nightclub. Lovers can go together, for that matter, to enjoy the entertainment and stimulants. Or, lacking a lover, one goes alone. There are many choices—things to suit different tastes. The decor is always charming, and conducive to pleasure. There are foyers and hallways that are museums of beautiful erotic art. Statues, paintings. I have my favorites—Hercules pleasuring Aphrodite, done in enormous white marble, every detail marvelously executed and visible. I like the warm-water, perfumed baths with their fountains and waterfalls and underwater lights. Of course, whenever there are dancing girls, I'm one of them (often the star). I can do everything from a Moulin Rouge can-can to a harem girl's gyrating belly dance, not to mention a tableau of naked statues come to life—Venus and Apollo, a nymph and a faun, consummating their desires in a ballroom that recreates a misty green forest. Couples can dance in many ways . . . costumed; naked; in dim light making love as they move to waltzes, tangos. There are rooms where a handsome, naked masseur pleasures me with massage . . . his skill matched by his enjoyment of his job. There is a large room where men and women walk about, exposing their bodies while they sip champagne. They fondle and examine each other in the manner of enjoying tasty canapes before a banquet. This is entertaining to me, because most of the men have erections—a room filled with erected penises is a dream room come to life. What fun to see so many shapes and sizes—to give one a little tweak, another a nice rub. . . . A certain type pleases me most. We all have our preferences. Occasionally, a man will slip one to me . . . right inside. Then I can tweak or rub him with other than my hand. We are a parade of beautiful bodies, engaged in little dancing and fondling movements. No ugliness here. No pot bellies, pendulous breasts, no wrinkled skin (cosmetic surgery corrects all those things by now; I think it was Marlene Dietrich who said, nudity is easy for the beautiful; difficult for the ugly). If one wants to grab a quick orgasm, one can, but there's more to come. Sometimes you just can't help getting carried away. Fulfillment is a delight at any given moment, titillating those who are not directly involved. I couldn't help myself for a moment there; he just popped it in while we were dancing, and we spilled champagne over my breasts (we got rather active and excited), so I think I'll go bathing. . . . The pool is languidly warm; I swim like a fish after playing in the cooling fountain. Beautiful men swim by me with erections like fish nosing into the crevices of my body. One pokes gently at my backside while another teases my pubes. The silhouettes of our bodies look graceful with the underwater lights shining. The lights turn rose, then blue, then green, then gold . . . then rose again. I spread my legs for the pleasant sensation of catching fish . . . my breasts are being stroked by wet slippery hands. Erections swim at me from every direction . . . I think I've caught a good one. He is strong enough to hold me above water while I squeeze his penis up inside me. The water froths and bubbles. The water has a delicious Jacuzzi movement—waves pulsing and lapping, inside and out. I'm a bit of a glutton, but this is one gluttony that never makes you fat. . . . Again . . . just hold it there another moment. I can hear applause. They applaud me, and I applaud myself. It's clever to be such a glutton . . . I could do it again and again . . . but then I'm not trying out for the Olympics or anything. Big deal. I'm just here to enjoy myself.

The invitation comes from a most interesting man—the impressario of my favorite Pleasure Place. He has a lot of style and is rather jaded. They say he has a special room where the most extraordinary things take place. Rumors are that he's so used to all this, it takes something quite beyond the ordinary to please him. He's a bit of a voyeur of course (but that's fun and allowed . . .). Looks a little bit like Humphrey Bogart . . . George Raft . . . Rudolph Valentino . . . and maybe Alonzo Cludish (he was twenty-first century, so anyone reading this, twentieth century, wouldn't know whom I was talking about), Marcello Mastroianni—of course, Marcello in 8½ would do quite well. . . . The impressario . . . this particular fellow . . . all jaded and Don Juanish, it is said, has a room where women come, and go out of their minds with desire. He has a machine, they say, where twenty-four-hour-orgasms are produced and used to write the most crashing symphonic music (his son, a composer-conductor of great genius takes credit). That is, you see, if he can drive a woman crazy enough in this room of his, the electronic impulses of her agony-ecstasy are reproduced in musical form. It's just a rumor, what he can do . . . but of course it's scientifically possible.

His invitation has nothing to do with music. It seems, on the surface, to be purely part of his own lucrative business. (He is the businessman, his son the genius. Sort of a Godfather thing. . . .) What he wants, he says, is that I become a giantess for a week or two. He can extend the cellular structure of my being (sexual and otherwise) to as great a degree as he wishes by the use of a new machine he has purchased. I can be enormous; mountains for breasts . . . a vagina like Carlsbad Caverns. . . .

I don't get it. . . . What's the point?

Men have never fulfilled their real sexual desires, he

explains. They dream of crawling about like hungry worm-babies in mountainous, squishy breasts . . . and then they would like to go further . . . be sucked into the soft, deep caverns of the womb. God knows, it was the best heaven they ever knew. . . . We've never been able to give anyone this opportunity before. The machine I bought for you cost me a billion.

Why me?

I've been watching you . . . when you come here to enjoy yourself.

He watches me with admiring, appreciative eyes. There is something fascinating about the dark wisdom of jaded, knowing eyes. I like them better than questioning, worried ones.

Watching me? (Little old me. . . .)

Yes, and I'm sure you'd really enjoy this, and I would enjoy your enjoying, and so could hundreds of others. Picture yourself . . . an enormous giantess. Your body a universe. Each man a phallic symbol. You are the sea, and they can swim in you. You are the moon rising above them. Your tremendous orgasms shake the earth. People would like to see that . . . feel the tremors. Can you imagine?

Something is missing, I say. Who could satisfy me now? A penis the size of the tip of a used toothpick? And can you picture how ugly my skin would be? Pores that would look gutted by the acne of meteorites. You ever see pores under a magnifying glass? I don't want to be a monster.

That would be a simple thing to correct with the machine. We can program it to make your skin as smooth as you wish. You will be entered by a team of scuba divers. Their equipment is not the clumsy old-fashioned kind that would be irritating and in the way. Think of it . . . penis-sized men struggling up into your depths—as many as would please you. You would be the first woman in history to experience orgasms by the entry of the entire body, and being, of a man into your tunnel of love. You can return to normal size anytime you wish.

Listen, I say, the contractions inside my vagina during orgasm might squeeze a poor little man to death. . . .

No, that's not possible. They would enjoy the sensation of your orgasm over their entire bodies—it would be a sexual rebirth.

First of all, on this night when I'm to become a giantess—the greatest sex goddess of all time—I get to pick the vaginal-astronauts of my choice. All fine specimens, muscular, strong-looking, possessing my favorite type of cocks. I choose more than I figure I'll need, just for the fun of choosing. Then, because there is no inside building large enough to contain a giantess, we go outside into a very lovely, starlit, moonlit night. We won't need any spotlights, I say. The moonlight is just perfect (I'm still a little worried about how my skin will look). I step inside the designated few acres of space and walk to the center. I'm wearing a lacy, push-up bra and little panties. Because on my body they are as much a part of my cellular structure as are my fingernails and hair, they will enlarge with me. The machine is beamed on me; its rays feel rather like a warm breeze. I can smell the faint odor of ozone produced by the tremendous rush of energy. I begin to grow, quite painlessly—a pulsing sensation. I am rising up toward the starry sky. It seems as close as a ceiling. The moon is a glowing light bulb. I can see for miles, lights and buildings, roads and mountains, rivers and seas. Down below me, hundreds of miniature people stare upward in wonder and awe. A big safety net is being quickly constructed on my acre of space (which seems only a few feet to me now). My squadron of deep-sea divers stand ready and waiting at its edge. They are naked except for suitably shaped helmets on their heads (like the reddish tips of penises—outsized to them, but now quite suitable to me—a six- or seven-foot man, the equivalent of a six- or seven-inch cock . . .). Dance music has been turned on over loudspeakers, but it is faint and far away to me. "Turn up the music, please," I say, and my voice, louder than any loudspeaker, reverberates over the landscape. The

Lilliputians below clasp their hands over their ears. The music is turned up, and I can hear the drumbeat. I sway to the rhythm. I am a beautiful giantess-sex-goddess. No one has ever seen anything like me before. I pull down one side of my bra, exposing a soft white mountain of a breast. I draw down the other side, and two heavy, mountain-breasts swing over the crowd, joggling as I dance. Some of the little men (overcome with the sight, it would seem) faint or collapse. I feel very heavy, but it is a pleasant, slow heaviness like slow-motion films. I have a beautiful, monstrous, symmetrical body. I put my fingers on the top of my panties and begin to push them down. I push them down to my thighs, exposing a naked, slowly gyrating pelvis of unbelievable size. Little heads crane upward. I can see their wide open eyes and mouths. I have to be careful when I draw up one leg (I'd hate to lose my balance and step on anybody). I pull my panties off, one leg and then the other, stand with my legs spread apart. "So, Little People . . ." I whisper very softly, although my voice still echoes from mountaintop to shining sea. "You've never seen anything like this before?" I rock my pelvis and spread my legs wider apart as I bend my knees. For a moment, my bed-sized clitoris is exposed above them. They jump up and down with excitement. "Let's see it again . . . again . . ." I can hear them crying in little voices like mewing kittens. "Please, Great Sex Goddess . . . show us again!" I fingertip my labia apart for a few seconds, smiling down on them. The moisture of my excitement creates drops of falling rain. Giant Goddesses do everything on a grand scale.

"Well, my cocky astronauts . . ." I whisper to my crew. "Are you ready for your journey?"

This starts a flurry among them. They scurry about under the safety net, carrying metal parts. In a minute, they've fashioned a towering (to them—only loin-high to me) erector-set stepladder between my legs; I watch them clamber up. The first and fastest cock-man reaches the top, and I pick him up and press his naked little body against one of my great breasts. He squirms and rubs himself into the flesh appreciatively. When I take him away from my breast, I see that his adorable toothpick-tip-sized prick is sticking straight up. "You darling little things you . . ." I whisper (loud as a foghorn) and ever so gently, hold him up to my mouth, licking him all over. His legs spread and kick delightedly in the air while my big wet tongue licks his loins and bottom. I fit his tiny cock like a pencil tip between my lips. He hangs on to my loose-hanging, twenty-foot-long hair, and I can hear little groans and moans coming from under his helmet while I suck as if his cock were a small straw, wriggling my tongue against it. In a few seconds, he collapses limply in my hand, and I can taste a few miniature drops of semen on my tongue. My other cock-men have reached the top of the ladder by now and are probing and examining my giant clitoris. It tickles quite pleasantly. I spread my legs to make the most of it. "Ummm . . ." I murmur echoingly. They certainly know their business. Some of them may have been special masseurs before this adventure. "Well . . ." I whisper to the limp one in my hand. "Do you want to go on with the others, or do you need a breather?" There are noises from under his helmet I can't quite hear. I put the phallic tip into my ear. "What did you say?"

"I said I want to go on. I'd like to be the first one in if I may. A big step for mankind, and myself as well!"

I repeat these brave words in a whisper for the crowd's benefit. They applaud—an oddly squeaky little sound. I put the cock-man back on the ladder top with the others. "He's first, remember. After all he got to the top of the ladder first."

His phallic-tip helmet enters my cavern smoothly. Then he seems to get a bit stuck, pushing hard with his feet against the ladder. He is a bit broad in the shoulders for a cock. I have to help a little—turning him this way and that until his shoulders work through. I can feel the pressure inside me of his squirming and pushing upward.

It is quite an extraordinary sensation. "Wow . . ." I say, forgetting the Lilliputians' delicate eardrums, but most of them are too wonderstruck and excited to bother covering their ears. They've all undressed by now and are empathetically imitating myself and the cock-men. The women with wide-spread legs and rocking hips; the men shuddering and wriggling as if trying to squirm into my body. My number one cock-man has disappeared, but I can feel him working inside me like crazy. By God, I can tell you, a broad-shouldered cock with arms and legs is something else!

The next one needs some assistance, too. I'm getting so steamy and ready, I shove him rather violently into me when he gets stuck. The two of them fill me up. If they keep wriggling like that, I'm going to come any minute. My torso is shaking all over the place. I jerk my hips, and my feet jump a little, shaking the ground. But now the second one has disappeared after a moment of legs sticking out and kicking. I do like to have something stretching apart the opening, rubbing my clitoris. I assist a third, as far as he'll go, which is just about right. Penis-head inside and broad shoulders where I need him outside. With the three of them overflowing my insides and moving like snakes or fish, I'm almost out of my mind. . . . It's going to be an orgasm to shake the earth; I hope I don't hurt anything . . . or any-one. . . . But I've gone this far, and it's going to have to come. . . . "Look out!" I say, like a crash of thunder. I dance wildly, and the world shudders and shakes. The moonbulb in the sky jiggles, and the stars whirl around. It's coming, and it's going to be big; oh, so sweet and big!

The first orgasm expels a cock-man like a ping-pong ball into the net. I don't stop, but just keep working at it, and the second jolt sends the second man whirling out like a trapeze artist. I've got one good one left . . . I can feel him moving from the depths of my insides like a hearty eel. I can't help screaming with the pleasure of this last one—shudders in my whole body that make trees sway and rocks come rolling down mountains. As I complete my giant orgasm, number one cock-man shoots forth from my inside Pleasure Place; his darling little prick is ejaculating a tiny fountain of semen into the air.

I sit down in my small space, a little out of breath, being careful not to disturb anything or squash anyone. The earth is still shaking. I see that my Lilliputians are having the orgy of their lives, and a few thousand orgasms—even in miniature—can create quite an earthquake.

The next night, I request that I be given a longer, larger area, because I think it would be great fun to have more cock-men, some of them rolling about and squirming and climbing over the soft flesh of my gigantic breasts, belly . . . while others take turns climbing up my great loin-crevice to dip themselves in and out of my soft red bathtub clitoris. This would have to be done while I'm lying down, stretched out to my full seventy-five or eighty feet. Then I can just lie there and feel them pushing themselves up into my cavern until the sensation drives me out of my mind. . . .

During the week that I was a Giant Sex Goddess, the impressario's son wrote some of the greatest symphonies of his career. As late as the twenty-third century, people were still going into orgasmic spasms just listening to them. . . . Then everybody got too jaded for that. Some rather extraordinary genital evolutionary changes had occurred . . . but then, that's another fantasy. . . .

AFTERWORD

☐ I have been able to print only a fraction of the letters I have received since publication of *My Secret Garden*. As I stated in the opening chapter, the overwhelming note of self-acceptance in these letters, the low level of guilt about sex, places this collection of material a generation ahead of those women who contributed to *Garden*.

In a sense, it took more courage for the women who appeared in my first book to talk about their fantasies. That was still a time when it was widely thought, even by therapists, that only "troubled" women had fantasies. The subject had not yet been given mass media okay, it had not been widely discussed on television, in newspapers and magazines.

The women who appear in these pages, above all, had the comfort of having read *My Secret Garden* before they wrote me. It helped them to look at themselves and their sexuality in a new light; it gave them information on the most intimate ideas and experiences of other women with which to compare themselves. As you have noticed, almost every letter contains the phrase, "Thank God, I'm not the only one."

But women's sexuality is only half the picture. If we believe in liberation, we must accept the logic that women cannot be free if our men are still chained to old, outworn, *macho* notions. If women are experts at sexual fantasy (as I believe we are), perhaps our outspokenness about it, our honesty about what we really think and feel will encourage men to reassess their sexual lives too.

Half the mail I have received since *Garden* has been from men. Most of them have been fascinated to find there was an aspect of female sexuality that up to now had been hidden or closed to them. I originally wanted to include these letters from men at the back of this volume. I thought it would be informative and exciting for women, but I thought men too would receive reinforcement, finding broader dimensions to their own sexuality. It was this latter idea—plus lack of space—that made me change my mind and go along with the suggestion so many men made in their letters: why not give male sexuality the space it deserved, and do a totally separate book on men's sexual fantasies?

If *Garden* had freed women to roam in wider sexual latitudes than they had believed possible or were capable of, it had also suggested to men that they too might be erotically more imaginative than their own literature and culture had so far depicted them. Any person reading *Garden*, or this book, can feel how liberating it is for a woman to know that even her most bizarre tastes and ideas are shared by other women. It is the compelling emotion of both books: "Thank God, I am not alone." I used to think men shared some mystic mass camaraderie, that simply being a man meant you belonged to "The Club." I have come to believe that many men, in their sexuality at least, are as hidden and lonely as we women have been.

The fact is, I don't know anything about men's sexual fantasies . . . except for the glimpse I've been given in the mail to date. The main thing it has taught me is that I have been wrong to assume that male eroticism was the simple stuff on which we were all raised: the films, magazines, advertisements, and so on, that depict men in our culture as compulsive consumers of the Penthouse Bunny, the man who can't get enough tits and ass, who dreams of devouring women like peanuts, and who doesn't feel sexual unless he's aggressive.

At the close of this book, there is an address where men can write me. I hope they will be as frank as the women whose letters we have just read, and will send in their fantasies—during sex, masturbation, and those that pop into the mind at all other times, too—for a forth-coming book. Please use the language which is natural to you, and include as much autobiographical detail as possible. What makes a fantasy most interesting and valuable to a researcher is an understanding of the life out of which it grows.

I expect to be surprised by what I receive. It is time that men too were released from the normative bludgeon-ing of the media that equates cowboys in cigarette ads with masculinity, and a cold heart with virility. If we have been surprised by the variety and extent of women's sexual imagination as seen through their fantasies, why should we not expect to find a new dimension in men's sexuality as well?

And if we do, won't both sexes be all the better for it? ☐

A LAST-MINUTE WORD FROM
NANCY FRIDAY

I am presently at work on a new book of women's sexual fantasies. If you would like to contribute, you may write to me at the address below. Please be as detailed as possible about the content of the fantasy; include age, marital status, family history plus any other autobiographical sexual history. As always, I guarantee your anonymity. Write:

NANCY FRIDAY
P.O. Box 1418
Washington, CT
06793

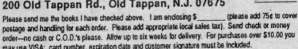